An introduction to radioimmunoassay
and related techniques

LABORATORY TECHNIQUES IN BIOCHEMISTRY AND MOLECULAR BIOLOGY

Edited by

T.S. WORK – *Cowes, Isle of Wight (formerly N.I.M.R., Mill Hill, London)*

E. WORK – *'East Lepe', 60 Solent View Road, Cowes, Isle of Wight*

Advisory board

P. BORST – *University of Amsterdam*
D.C. BURKE – *University of Warwick*
P.B. GARLAND – *University of Dundee*
M. KATES – *University of Ottawa*
W. SZYBALSKI – *University of Wisconsin*
H.G. WITTMAN – *Max-Planck Institut für Molekulaire Genetik, Berlin*

ELSEVIER BIOMEDICAL PRESS
AMSTERDAM • NEW YORK • OXFORD

AN INTRODUCTION TO RADIOIMMUNOASSAY AND RELATED TECHNIQUES

T. Chard

Professor of Reproductive Physiology, Departments of Obstetrics, Gynaecology, and Reproductive Physiology, St. Bartholomew's Hospital Medical College and the London Hospital Medical College, London, U.K.

ELSEVIER BIOMEDICAL PRESS
AMSTERDAM · NEW YORK · OXFORD

ISBN — series: 0 7204 4200 1
— paperback: 0-444-80424-2

First edition 1978
Second printing 1981
Second, completely revised edition 1982
Second printing 1985
Third printing 1986

Published by:

ELSEVIER BIOMEDICAL PRESS
1 MOLENWERF, P.O. BOX 211
1014 AG AMSTERDAM, THE NETHERLANDS

Sole distributors for the U.S.A. and Canada:

ELSEVIER-NORTH HOLLAND INC.
52 VANDERBILT AVENUE
NEW YORK, N.Y. 10017

Library of Congress Cataloging in Publication Data

Chard, T.
    An introduction to radioimmunoassay and related
techniques.

    (Laboratory techniques in biochemistry and molecular
biology)
    Bibliography: p.
    Includes index.
    1. Radioimmunoassay. 2. Immunoassay. I. Title.
II. Series. [DNLM: 1. Radioimmunoassay. W1 LA232K
v.6 pt.2 / QW 570 C471i]
QP519.9.R3C45 1982   574.1'9285   82-16397
ISBN 0-444-80420-X
ISBN 0-444-80424-2 (pbk.)

This book is the second edition of Volume 6, Part II, of the series 'Laboratory Techniques in Biochemistry and Molecular Biology'

Printed in The Netherlands

Contents

Chapter 7. Requirements for binding assays – extraction of ligand from biological fluids, and collection and storage of samples . . . 143

Chapter 8. Requirements for binding assays – calculation of results 161

Chapter 9. Characteristics of binding assays – sensitivity 169

Chapter 10. Characteristics of binding assays – specificity 185

Chapter 11. Characteristics of binding assays – precision. 203

Chapter 12.   Characteristics of binding assays – relation to other types of assay.   223

Chapter 13.   Automation of binding assays   233

Chapter 14.   Organisation of assay services   243

Appendices

List of abbreviations

RIA	= radioimmunoassay		^{125}I	= iodine 125
IRMA	= immunoradiometric assay		^{131}I	= iodine 131
EIA	= enzymoimmunoassay		cpm	= counts per minute
IEMA	= immunoenzymatic assay		dps	= disintegrations per second
FIA	= fluoroimmunoassay		FITC	= fluorescein isothiocyanate
IFMA	= immunofluorometric assay		PPO	= 2,5-diphenyloxazole
LIA	= luminescence immunoassay		POPOP	= 1,4-di-2(5-phenyloxazolyl)-benzene
CPB	= competitive protein binding			
RRA	= radioreceptor assay		pH	= hydrogen ion concentration
Ag	= antigen		V	= volts
Ab	= antibody		Log_e	= natural logarithm
AgAB	= antigen–antibody complex		v/v	= volume by volume
k_1	= forward association constant		w/v	= weight by volume
k_2	= reverse association constant		hPL	= human placental lactogen
B	= bound fraction		hGH	= human growth hormone
F	= free fraction		ACTH	= adrenocorticotrophic hormone
b	= proportion of tracer bound as % of that in zero standard		LH	= luteinizing hormone
μg	= microgram		FSH	= follicle-stimulating hormone
ng	= nanogram		TSH	= thyroid-stimulating hormone
pg	= picogram		AVP	= arginine-vasopressin
fg	= femtogram		LVP	= lysine-vasopressin
nm	= nanometre		hCG	= human chorionic gonadotrophin
μ	= micron			
mol	= mole		AFP	= alpha-fetoprotein
nmol	= nanomole		CEA	= carcino-embryonic antigen
M	= molar		T_3	= triiodothyronine
mM	= millimolar		T_4	= thyroxine
M_r	= relative molecular mass		CBG	= cortisol-binding globulin
Ci	= Curie		TBG	= thyroxine-binding globulin
mCi	= milliCurie		SHBG	= sex-hormone-binding globulin
μCi	= microCurie			
^{3}H	= tritium		LATS	= long-acting thyroid stimulator
^{14}C	= carbon 14			

AMP	= adenosine monophosphate	IgG	= immunoglobulin G
ATP	= adenosine triphosphate	DNP	= dinitrophenol
NAD	= nicotinamide adenine dinucleotide	ANS	= anilino napthalene sulphonic acid
$PGF_{2\alpha}$	= prostaglandin $F_{2\alpha}$	KIU	= kallikrein inhibitor units
FgD	= fragment D of fibrinogen	WHO	= World Health Organisation
FgE	= fragment E of fibrinogen		

CHAPTER 1

The background to radioimmunoassay

1.1. Introduction

The introduction of radioimmunoassay (Yalow and Berson, 1960) is probably the single most important advance in biological measurement of the past two decades. Together with related techniques it has revolutionised one major discipline — endocrinology — and has exerted a similar influence in other fields, notably haematology, pharmacology, and cancer detection. This success can be attributed to three factors.

(1) It has many advantages when compared with previous methods; for instance, in the case of a hormone, the gain in sensitivity, specificity, and ease of performance over a classical biological assay.

(2) It can be applied to substances for which there was no previous assay method.

(3) Perhaps most importantly radioimmunoassay and related techniques offer a general system for the measurement of an immensely wide range of materials.

Thus, a technician skilled in the radioimmunoassay of a protein such as growth hormone would find little difficulty, either conceptual or in terms of equipment required, in setting up a comparable assay for a steroid hormone such as cortisol, a drug such as digoxin, or a cancer product such as carcino-embryonic antigen.

The aim of this book is to set out the basic concepts of radioimmunoassay and related techniques in such a way as to assist those who are embarking on the subject for the first time, or who already have some practical experience but are seeking to broaden their knowledge of the subject as a whole. It does not set out to provide an exhaustive review, which would now be impossible with the size and rapid growth of the subject, or to provide detailed recipes for individual assays. Instead, an attempt will be made to underline the common ground in all assays of this type, whether it be in the preparation of materials, the use of these materials or the interpretation of results. Specific examples, where they are used, are always intended to illustrate the general rather than the particular.

1.2. Terminology

It is necessary at an early stage to define some terms which will recur throughout the book. All techniques involve the combination of two materials, one of which is referred to as the 'binder' and the other as the 'ligand'; the substance measured, which could be binder or ligand, is referred to as the 'analyte'. The terms are valuable because radioimmunoassay is only one, albeit the most widely applied, of a series of related techniques. The term which best embraces the whole field is 'binding assays': this signifies any procedure in which quantitation of a material depends on the progressive saturation of a specific binder by that material, and the subsequent determination of its distribution between 'bound' and 'free' phases. This general principle can include many different binders and many different methods for determining the distribution between the bound and free phases (Table 1.1). The most familiar subdivisions of binding assays are based on the nature of the binder employed: 'immunoassays' where this is an antibody; 'competitive protein binding assay' where this is a naturally occurring binding protein; and 'receptor assay' where the binder is a naturally occurring cell receptor. Determination of the distribution between bound and free phases usually depends on physicochemical separation of these phases, the distribution being followed by the incorporation of a 'tracer' consisting of a small amount of the ligand labelled with a radioactive isotope. However, neither of these features are implicit in the definition of a binding assay. For instance, it is possible to use labelled binder as tracer rather than labelled ligand; this is the 'immunometric' assay*. The label does not have to be a radioisotope: it can

---

* It has been suggested that radioimmunoassays (labelled antigen) can be described as 'limited reagent' methods, and immunoradiometric assays (labelled antibody) as 'reagent excess' methods. However, this is not a logical distinction, since radioimmunoassays can be conducted with an excess of tracer (e.g. in late addition systems), and immunoradiometric assays with a limiting amount of tracer.

TABLE 1.1
The place of radioimmunoassay and related techniques among assays for biological
materials

The three basic procedures are biological, physicochemical, and binding assays.
'Binding' assays may be directed at the measurement of binder or ligand. In assays
for the ligand, three different types of binder are available, which in principle may
be used with any of the six types of tracer shown. With any combination of these
the final step may separate bound and free ligand, or bound and free binder, or may
not require any separation

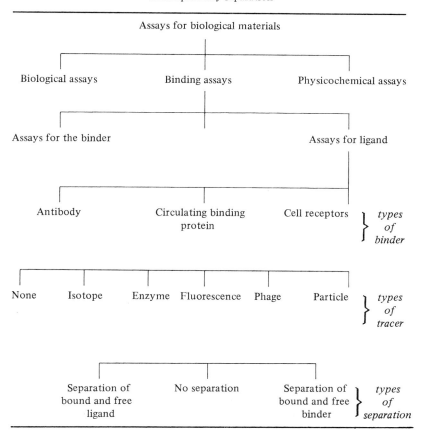

equally be any material which can be measured precisely in very small quantities, such as a fluorescent compound (fluoroimmunoassay, FIA), or an enzyme (enzymoimmunoassay, EIA). Finally, the separation of the phases is not always essential: if the characteristics of the tracer in the bound and free phases are sufficiently different then no separation is necessary.

1.3. Early development of radioimmunoassay

Recent discussion of the history of binding assays has been marred by claims and counter-claims for priority in the development of the technique. This may be expected in any subject which expands far beyond the expectations of its originators. The argument will not be described in detail here but a simple and doubtless equally arguable conclusion will be put forward: that a technique using an antibody as the binder (i.e. radioimmunoassay) was first described by Yalow and Berson in the USA (Yalow and Berson, 1960); and that a technique using a naturally occurring binding protein (i.e., competitive binding assay) was described by Ekins in the U.K. (Ekins, 1960).

For a full historical perspective one must look back further than the original description of individual methods. It is noteworthy that the first techniques were developed in laboratories of nuclear medicine. The common thread was the ability to handle radioactive isotopes, which in turn had become available for routine biomedical use as a by-product of the development of nuclear weapons. The striking feature of many radioactive isotopes is that the energy of their emission is so great that it becomes possible to detect even a few atoms with relatively simple equipment. When such atoms are attached to another molecule, then the latter can be detected in equally small numbers. In practice, it was probably the ability to measure very small quantities of a tracer compound, rather than an appreciation of the potential use of antibodies and other binders of high affinity, which led to the original development of radioimmunoassay. Claims for the originality of the concept of the technique must go back much further since it is, in essence, a combination of Archimedes principle and the Law of Mass Action.

The work of Yalow and Berson arose from their earlier studies on the behaviour of ^{131}I-labelled proteins in vivo; at the time (the early 1950's) this was a new and highly effective approach to the study of protein metabolism. One of the materials studied was ^{131}I-labelled insulin; this led to the demonstration that insulin-requiring diabetics almost always have a circulating insulin-binding protein (Berson et al., 1956). They also showed that the tracer could be displaced from the binder by large quantities of unlabelled insulin, and that the binding of the tracer was quantitatively related to the total amount of insulin present. These observations formed the basis of the first radioimmunoassay for insulin (see Yalow and Berson, 1971). However, the sensitivity of the assay using antibodies from the sera of insulin-treated diabetics was inadequate for the measurement of the relatively low circulating levels of endogenous human insulin. The next step, therefore, was the preparation of specific antisera to human insulin in guinea-pigs; this resulted in the first radioimmunoassay capable of detecting endogenous insulin in human blood (Yalow and Berson, 1960).

While this work was in progress, Ekins in the U.K. was examining the use of thyroxine-binding globulin for the measurement of thyroxine in human plasma. Together with techniques for vitamin B_{12} using intrinsic factor as the binding substance, these studies underlie all subsequent work on circulating binding protein assays.

1.4. Basic principles of binding assays

The basic principles of binding assays are simple once grasped. However, the newcomer is not helped by the fact that almost every writer on the subject has their own way of explaining the principles and that in the course of the explanation they are likely to denigrate the views of others as oversimplified or even positively in error. Much of the argument is semantic, since all are looking at the same basic system with the same basic endpoints.

For the sake of simplicity, it will be assumed here that the technique under discussion is a radioimmunoassay, i.e. using an antibody as the binder and an antigen as the ligand. The same principles, however, apply to any of the other systems which come under the heading of binding assays. A simple illustration of the mechanism of a radioimmunoassay is presented in Fig. 1.1 which shows binding of antigen to a fixed amount

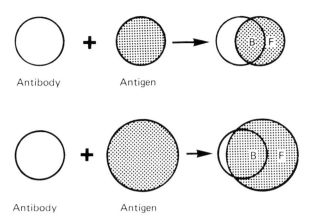

Fig. 1.1. The basic principle of a binding assay, using immunoassay as an example. If given amounts of antigen and antibody are allowed to react together (above) then at equilibrium they will form an antigen-antibody complex (the overlapping area B) together with a proportion of both the antibody and the antigen (F) which remain free. If the amount of antibody is held constant while the total amount of antigen is increased (below) then at equilibrium the amount of antigen–antibody complex (B) is increased; however, the increase in the free fraction (F) is relatively greater and thus yields a lower bound to free ratio.

of antibody in the presence of different total amounts of antigen. The distribution of the antigen between the bound and free phases is directly related to the total amount of antigen present and this provides a means for quantitating the latter.

Another approach to understanding the principle is through consideration of reversible reactions. As a starting point, consider the reversible reaction between an antigen and an antibody to form the antigen–antibody complex:

$$Ag + Ab \quad \underset{k_2}{\overset{k_1}{\rightleftharpoons}} \quad Ag\,Ab \tag{1.1}$$

In this equation, the rate constant of the forward reaction (association of antigen and antibody to form a complex) is denoted by k_1, and the rate constant of the reverse reaction (dissociation of the antigen–antibody complex) is denoted by k_2. It should be noted that k_1 and k_2 are *constants*, in other words they describe the *fraction* of the available molecules which will react within unit time. The absolute rate – the number of molecules which react in unit time – is obviously dependent on the concentration of molecules. Thus, when the reaction begins with the addition of antigen and antibody, the forward reaction rate is high and the reverse reaction rate correspondingly low:

$$Ag + Ab \ \rightleftarrows \ AgAb \tag{1.2}$$

As the reaction proceeds, the concentration of free Ag and Ab decreases, and so too will the forward reaction rate. At the same time the concentration of the antigen–antibody complex increases, and with it the rate of the reverse reaction. Eventually the stage is reached where the number of free Ag and Ab molecules reacting in unit time to form AgAb is identical with the number of AgAb molecules which dissociate in this time:

$$Ag + Ab \ \rightleftharpoons \ AgAb \tag{1.3}$$

At this stage of equilibrium there will be no further net change in the concentration of the molecules on the two sides of the equation. In most, but not all, radioimmunoassay systems the reagents are permitted to react for long enough for equilibrium to be reached and eq. (1.3) can therefore be used as the basis for further discussion.

The exact concentrations which are reached at equilibrium will depend on the energy with which the binder and ligand react. In thermodynamic terminology, this can be described as ΔS, or the change in free energy within the system as a whole. The situation can be described by the Law of Mass Action which states that, at equilibrium, the ratio of the products of the concentrations on the two sides of the equation will be constant, designated as K:

$$\frac{[AgAb]}{[Ag][Ab]} = K \tag{1.4}$$

where [Ag], [Ab] and [AgAb] are the concentrations of free antigen, free antibody and antigen–antibody complex, respectively, and K is the affinity constant*. Since the final concentrations are determined by the rate constants of the forward and reverse reactions it is also apparent that:

$$K = \frac{k_1}{k_2} \qquad (1.5)$$

The affinity constant, K, for any system provides a measure of the energy of reaction between the original reagents, in this case Ag and Ab. Given fixed starting concentrations, a high K value would imply that at equilibrium the concentration of the Ag Ab complex will be much greater than that of free Ag and Ab, while a low K value would imply the reverse situation.

Assume a system of given K value, that the initial molar concentration of Ag and Ab are equal, and that these concentrations are chosen so that at equilibrium both Ag and Ab will be equally distributed between the bound and free phases. Let us also assume that the starting concentration of each reagent is 2 (which could be in any concentration units). At equilibrium:

$$\underset{1}{Ag} + \underset{1}{Ab} \; \rightleftharpoons \; \underset{1}{Ag\,Ab} \qquad (1.6)$$

Looking at the antigen alone, 1 unit is bound and 1 unit is free. Now take the system but with 4 units of Ag rather than 2. It follows from the Law of Mass Action that an increase in the concentration of reactants on one side of the equation will produce a corresponding increase on the other side, i.e. an increase in Ag or Ab, or both will produce an increase in the concentration of Ag Ab at equilibrium. But in the case described, the in-

---

* The units of K are litres per mole (1/mol) which can be confusing to the uninitiated. It arises from the fact that K is derived by dividing a concentration (mol/1) by the product of two other concentrations, that is:

$$\frac{mol/1}{mol/1 \times mol/1} = \frac{1}{mol/1} = 1/mol$$

In immunoassay the terms 'affinity' and 'avidity' are often used interchangeably. It has been suggested that 'affinity' should be used to describe the properties of the antigen and 'avidity' the properties of the antibody.

crease in Ag Ab cannot be equivalent to that in Ag, because Ab has remained unchanged. Thus, although the concentration of Ag Ab will increase, that of free Ag will increase relatively more. For the sake of illustration, some entirely hypothetical figures may be given to this situation:

$$\underset{2.8}{Ag} + \underset{0.8}{Ab} \rightleftharpoons \underset{1.2}{Ag\,Ab} \qquad (1.7)$$

Looking again at the antigen alone, 1.2 units are bound, but 2.8 units are free. In the situation of eq. (1.6), the ratio of bound to free antigen at equilibrium was 1. The addition of more antigen has decreased this ratio to 0.43.

A conclusion may now be drawn:
GIVEN AN UNVARYING QUANTITY OF BINDER OF FIXED K VALUE, THE RATIO OF BOUND TO FREE LIGAND AT EQUILIBRIUM WILL BE QUANTITATIVELY RELATED TO THE TOTAL AMOUNT OF LIGAND PRESENT.
This is the basic principle of all binding assays.

The concepts of tracer, of standards, and of the separation of bound and free phases have not yet been introduced because all of these are secondary to the underlying principle, and not defining features. For example, in most if not all cases, the labelled ligand should be identical with the unlabelled ligand and should behave identically in combination with the binder. Under these circumstances the eventual distribution between bound and free phases will be determined by the total amount of ligand present and not independently by the amount of labelled or unlabelled ligand. The tracer is incorporated simply because it provides a technically convenient means for measuring the distribution of bound and free; the irrelevance of tracer ligand to the basic principle is illustrated by the fact that it is equally possible to use the binder as the tracer (see § 6.4). Following on these arguments, the use of the term 'competition', which is frequently used to describe the relationship between labelled and unlabelled ligand, should be discouraged. In most binding assays both have equal opportunities for combination with the binder, and the final result depends on the total number of ligand molecules present.

Standards — a series of different concentrations of purified ligand against which the results of unknowns can be judged — are again a technical convenience. Given a knowledge of the exact concentrations of tracer and binder, and the K value, the concentration of an unknown could be determined by simple calculation without the need for reference to standards. In practice, however, the vagaries of reagents are such that this hypothetical situation cannot be achieved. Finally, the separation of the bound and free phases is yet another technical manoeuvre unrelated to the basic principle: systems have been described in which it is unnecessary.

1.5. Binder dilution curves and standard curves

The discussion of principles will now be extended to the two basic experimental procedures of saturation analysis – the setting up of binder dilution curves and of standard curves.

The binder dilution curve (or antibody dilution curve in the context of a radioimmunoassay) involves the incubation of a fixed amount of tracer ligand with different concentrations of the binder; for example, serial doubling dilutions of an antiserum. Following incubation, the distribution of the tracer in the bound and free fractions is ascertained. The general appearance of this type of curve is shown in Fig. 1.2. Plotted as percentage of tracer bound against serial dilutions of the binder on a logarithmic scale the curve is sigmoidal. Given a suitable set of reagents, the construction of this curve is the first step in setting up a binding assay system, since the results may determine the amount of binder for use in a standard curve.

As a rule of thumb, the concentration of binder chosen for use in a standard curve will be that which is sufficient to bind approximately 50% of tracer (Fig. 1.2). Exceptions to this rule will be discussed in later sections. At this concentration, at which the amount of binder is sufficient to fix only half of the tracer, it is apparent that the addition of further ligand must lead to a substantially greater increase in the free fraction than the bound fraction. By contrast, if a much higher concentration of binder is chosen (e.g., 2.5 in Fig. 1.2) the amount of ligand required to produce a significant shift in the bound and free fractions will be much greater, and the eventual assay less sensitive.

The standard curve involves the incubation of fixed amounts of tracer ligand and binder with different concentrations of unlabelled ligand.

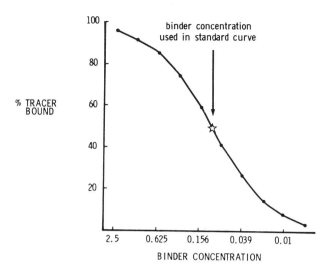

Fig. 1.2. A binder dilution curve (e.g., an antibody dilution curve). Serial dilutions of the binder (horizontal axis) are incubated with a fixed amount of tracer ligand, and the percentage of the latter bound plotted on the vertical axis. In a typical binding assay the amount of binder chosen is that which will bind 50% of the tracer; however, there are many exceptions to this. The example shown is derived from a theoretical model of a binding assay (see § 1.9).

Plotted as the percentage of tracer bound against serial dilutions of the ligand on a logarithmic scale this again gives a sigmoid curve (Fig. 1.3). At the upper end of this curve, the small quantities of unlabelled ligand produce minor shifts in the distribution between the bound and free phases. At the lower end of the curve, the total concentration of ligand relative to that of the binder is such that the majority is in the free form. Between these two extremes is a range of ligand concentrations at which relatively small changes produce a significant alteration in the distribution of bound and free. For the situation shown in Fig. 1.3 this range would be from 0.032–2. In practical terms this, the steepest part of the slope, represents the effective range of the assay.

The standard curve is the basic requirement for quantitation of the

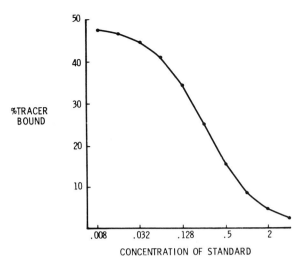

Fig. 1.3. A standard curve. Fixed amounts of tracer ligand and binder (the latter at the concentration shown in Fig. 1.2) are incubated with varying concentrations of standard unlabelled ligand (horizontal axis). The percentage of the tracer bound (vertical axis) is progressively reduced with increasing concentrations of standard. Note from Fig. 1.1 that the *total* amount of ligand bound (tracer plus standard) is actually increased as the *proportion* of ligand bound is decreased. The horizontal axis is also sometimes referred to as the 'dose metameter' and the vertical axis as the 'response metameter'.

ligand in unknown samples. When the sample is substituted for the standard, and using the same fixed concentrations of binder and tracer, the value determined for the distribution of the bound and free phases will be equivalent to some value on the horizontal scale of the standard curve. This value can be read by simple extrapolation (Fig. 1.4).

Practical techniques for setting up binder dilution curves and standard curves are shown in Tables 1.2 and 1.3 and Fig. 1.5–1.7. It must be emphasised again that these, together with all other detailed technical descriptions in the book, are intended as examples. The potential range of variations, including buffers used, volumes, time of incubation and temperature, is enormous. Some of these variations will have little effect on the results obtained; others, for example order of addition of reagents, may have dramatic effects which are considered in later chapters.

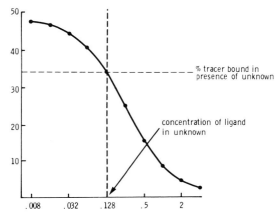

Fig. 1.4. Estimation of the amount of ligand in an unknown sample using a standard curve. The conditions are identical with those shown in Fig. 1.3. The unknown sample is incubated with the same fixed concentrations of binder and tracer, and the percentage of tracer bound is approximately 34%; this corresponds to a value of 0.128 for the standards, and this is therefore the concentration in the unknown. Note that where duplicate determinations are performed, it is customary to take the mean of the two counts, and to use this mean for subsequent calculation. It is not good practice to make separate potency estimates from the two replicates, and then to take the mean of these.

TABLE 1.2
Construction of a binder dilution curve
(Radioimmunoassay of human placental lactogen, hPL)

Diluent buffer : 0.05 M phosphate (pH 7.5) containing 2 mg/ml bovine serum albumin (see Table 1.4 for buffer preparations)

1. Prepare serial doubling dilutions of an antiserum to hPL in 1 ml of diluent buffer (see Fig. 1.5 and 1.6). The range to be covered will vary between different antisera, but typically would be 1 : 100 − 1 : 100,000.
2. Dispense 0.25 ml of each dilution into duplicate tubes; include one pair containing diluent buffer with no antiserum to act as an assay blank.
3. To each tube add 0.2 ml of a solution of ^{125}I-labelled hPL, diluted such that the total counts per tube are approximately 10,000−15,000 in 10 sec. Include one pair of tubes containing tracer alone for measurement of total counts.
4. To each tube add 0.05 ml of serum or plasma from a non-pregnant adult, or a non-human species such as the cow or horse.
5. Incubate for 1 h at room temperature.

6. Add 1 ml of a 20% solution of polyethylene glycol and proceed as shown in Table 6.3.
7. Place the tube in the well crystal of a γ-counter and count for 10 sec.
8. Plot the results as % of tracer bound on the vertical axis against the dilution of antiserum on a log scale on the horizontal axis (see Fig. 1.2). Always plot both duplicates at each point.

Comments: The procedure outlined has been chosen arbitrarily from among an immense range of potential variations, all of which are likely to make little difference to the end result. However, some general comments can be made about the individual steps.

(*i*)   As a point of good practice, a series of 'master' dilutions are made (volume 1 ml) from which aliquots are then dispensed into the incubation tubes; this is much preferable to making 2 sets of doubling dilutions in 0.25 ml.
(*ii*) The volume chosen (0.25 ml) is based on two factors: achieving a final incubation volume of 0.5 ml; and doing this with volumes of the individual reagents which can be accurately and precisely dispensed from widely available equipment. Any other convenient volumes could be used (e.g., 0.05 ml antibody and 0.4 ml tracer) provided that the final concentrations are correctly recorded. With current equipment, pipetting precision of 1% or less can easily be obtained with any volume from 0.05 ml upwards.
(*iii*) The same observations on volume apply to the tracer. The choice of the total amount of tracer added, and the counting time required, will vary extremely widely according to the substance involved. The principles for selection of this quantity are discussed in § 9.2 and § 9.3.
(*iv*) The volume of serum chosen is based on the decision that this shall make up 10% of the total incubation volume. Smaller volumes may be difficult to dispense with a high degree of precision; large volumes may yield non-specific effects (§ 10.3).
(*v*)   As with other variations, the possible range of times and temperature is immense. In the early development of a new assay these factors should be investigated in detail, beginning with curves incubated for 1, 4, 24 and 48 h, at 4°C, room temperature and 37°C. Longer incubation times should be particularly examined in those systems in which high sensitivity is a requirement.
(*vi*) Almost all separation procedures can and have been applied to hPL (see table 6.1). The polyethylene glycol method has been chosen for its efficiency and simplicity.
(*vii*) It is not recommended that total counts are estimated for every tube. This will only show pipetting errors with the tracer; similar but sometimes more serious errors with the other reagents are not revealed.

Note: Because most commerical RIA kits for hPL contain an excess of antibody (in order to desensitise the system) they can be used as part of a class exercise in setting up binder dilution curves.

TABLE 1.3

Construction of standard curve

(Radioimmunoassay of human placental lactogen, hPL)

Diluent buffer: As for Table 1.2

1. Prepare standards of hPL in hPL-free serum or plasma, using a master standard containing 1 mg/ml (see Table 2.1).
2. Dispense 0.05 ml of each dilution into duplicate tubes; include two pairs containing hPL-free serum alone to act as assay blank and '0' standard (Fig. 1.7) and further duplicate tubes containing serum or plasma from subjects in late pregnancy. Always use the identical procedure and pipettes for sample and standards.
3. To each tube add 0.2 ml of a solution of ^{125}I-labelled hPL, diluted such that the total counts per tube are approximately 10,000–15,000 in 10 sec. Include one pair of tubes containing tracer alone for measurement of total counts.
4. To each tube add 0.25 ml of a 1 : 500 dilution of antiserum to hPL; in the case of the assay blank tubes add 0.25 ml diluent buffer in place of this.
5. Stand for 1 h at room temperature.
6. Add 1 ml of a solution of 20% polyethylene glycol and proceed as shown in Table 6.3.
7. Count each precipitate.
8. Plot the results as % tracer bound on the vertical axis against the concentration of standard on a log scale on the horizontal axis (see Fig. 1.3).
9. Calculate the results of unknowns as shown in Fig. 1.4.

Comments: The procedure outlined has been chosen arbitrarily from among an immense range of potential variations, many of which have already been discussed (see *Comments* to Table 1.2). Note that the choice of a 1 : 500 dilution of antiserum is arbitrary and would obviously have to be tested and varied with each different antiserum used. The dilution of antiserum appropriate to this type of desensitised assay represents a relative excess of antiserum and cannot, therefore, be extrapolated from the binder dilution curve (see § 9.3).

1.6. *Methods for plotting the standard curve*

The convention followed here (Fig. 1.3) is a semi-logarithmic plot of percentage tracer bound against the concentration of unlabelled ligand. This is a popular type of presentation, but there are many other ways of showing the same data. For the independent variable, there is only one commonly used alternative, an arithmetic scale of standard concentrations. Substitution of the latter in the percentage bound plot yields the

TABLE 1.4

Buffers for use in radioimmunoassay

A wide range of buffers has been used in radioimmunoassay. With very few exceptions the exact nature of the buffer is irrelevant provided it meets the following criteria:
1. pH within 1 unit of neutrality (i.e., pH 6−8)*;
2. Molarity in the range 0.01−0.1;
3. Freedom from organisms;
4. Freedom from contamination with ligand**.

Buffers are usually made up in distilled or de-ionised water; in most parts of the world tap water would be equally satisfactory though a more stringent specification would suggest that conductance should be less than 1 $\mu\Omega$. The composition of three commonly used buffers is given here, together with a note of some commonly used additives (Table 1.5). In some commercial kits dyes are added to aid identification, e.g., blue for antibody and yellow for tracer, yielding green in the final mixture.

Buffer	M_r	Amount (g/l)
Phosphate (pH 7.4)		
$Na_2HPO_4 \cdot 12 H_2O$	358.22	14.5
$Na H_2PO_4 \cdot 2 H_2O$	156.03	1.48
Tris (pH 8.0)		
Tris(hydroxymethyl) aminomethane	121.14	6.07
Titrate to pH 8.0 with 1 M HCl		
(approx. 29 ml)		
Barbiturate (pH 7.6)		
Sodium diethylbarbiturate	206.18	10.3
Titrate to pH 7.6 with 1 M HCl		
(approx. 33 ml)		

The pH of a buffer should always be checked after preparation, using either a
  pH meter or narrow-range indicator sticks (Neutralit, Merck).

* Steroid immunoassays can be remarkably independent of pH, working perfectly well at pH 3.5 (Rolleri et al., 1976)
** A routine and apparently simple assay occasionally goes dramatically wrong because of contamination of one of the basic reagents with ligand. A few crystals of purified material can turn a 20 l container of distilled water into a potent standard solution

TABLE 1.5

Common additives to buffer used in radioimmunoassay

Material	Source	Concentration	Purpose
Proteins such as:			
Bovine serum albumin*	Armour Pharmaceutical Company	1–10 mg/ml	To prevent absorption losses on to surface of tubes, and to stabilise proteins and peptides
Sodium azide	–	0.2–1 mg/ml	Bacteriostat
Merthiolate	E. Lilly and Company	0.1 mg/ml	Bacteriostat
Trasylol	Bayer Pharmaceuticals	1000 KIU**/ml	Inhibitor of trypsin-like enzymes (Zysnar, 1981)
Calcium salts	–	0.005 M	Enhance activity of certain antisera
Triton X-100 or other polyoxyethylenes	Rohm and Haas Company	0.1–1% (v/v)	Aids dispersion in solid phase systems; aids decantation in separation of bound and free phases

* Batches of purified proteins for use in radioimmunoassay should be checked for enzyme activity (which may lead to proteolysis of a tracer with corresponding reduction in the '0' standard) and for the presence of endogenous ligand (particularly with materials which are not species specific such as thyroxine and cortisol). To do this, standard curves should be set up containing the new batch of protein, and the results compared with those from a previous and satisfactory batch of protein (see Flatt, 1980). For removal of ligand, see Table 2.2

** Kallikrein inhibitor units

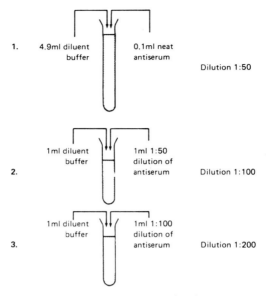

Fig. 1.5. Preparation of doubling dilutions of antiserum (see Table 1.2).

standard curve shown in Fig. 1.8. For the dependent variable, by contrast, there are many possible alternatives. The most popular is to use the ratio of bound to free ligand; Fig. 1.9 and 1.10 show this in arithmetic and logarithmic form. The inverse ratio, free to bound, can also be used (Fig. 1.11 and 1.12). A common variation on the percentage bound plot

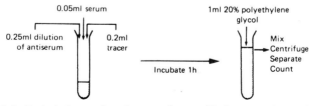

Fig. 1.6. Technical procedure for an antiserum dilution curve (see Table 1.2).

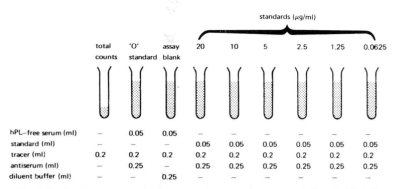

Fig. 1.7. Setting up a standard curve and appropriate controls (see Table 1.3).

is to express the results as a percentage of the distribution observed in the zero standard (i.e., a tube containing fixed amounts of tracer and binder, but no unlabelled ligand; this is also sometimes referred to as the 'antibody blank') (Fig. 1.13). Finally, the response variable may be described by several transformations of which the best known is the logit transformation (Rodbard and Lewald, 1970):

$$\text{logit } b = \log_e \left(\frac{b}{100 - b} \right) \qquad (1.8)$$

where b is the proportion of tracer bound expressed as a percentage of that in the zero standard. This type of plot has the advantage that in some, but not all, situations it gives a straight line rather than a curve (Fig. 1.14), thus simplifying calculation (see also § 8.3).

The choice of plot is very much a matter of the personal taste or past experience of the individual worker. Good arguments can be put forward for and against all the types described. A graph of percentage bound against log dose (Fig. 1.3) has the advantage that it directly reflects the output from the tracer detection system. Thus, in the case of a radioimmunoassay, if counts per minute is substituted for percentage bound, the shape of the curve would be identical. It is possible to see, at a glance, whether an apparent difference between two standard points is likely to be experimentally significant. This is not the case in the type of plot shown in

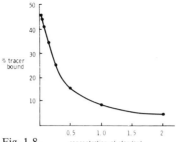

Fig. 1.8.

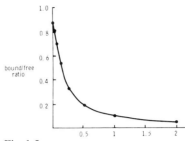

Fig. 1.9.

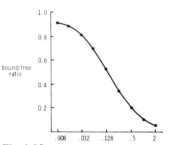

Fig. 1.10.

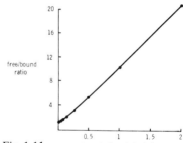

Fig. 1.11.

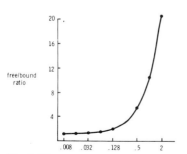

Fig. 1.12.

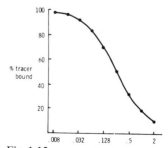

Fig. 1.13.

Fig. 1.13. By describing all points in relation to the zero standard, it may conceal problems from the uninitiated; for instance that the true percentage bound in the zero standard is less than 20%, and thus that the precision of all subsequent points must be highly suspect. The plot of bound/free ratio against log dose (Fig. 1.10), yields a curve very similar to that of percentage tracer bound. By contrast, the plot of free/bound ratio against log dose (Fig. 1.12) has a completely different appearance, and the important disadvantage that the slope at the various parts of the curve is quite unrelated to the experimental findings. It is accepted that it presents data identical to that of other plots; nonetheless, to the unwary who may associate steepness of slope with precision, it would seem that the effective range of the assay lies between standard concentrations of 0.5 and 2. A glance at the other plots clearly shows that this is not the case.

Plots using an arithmetic scale of standard concentrations again have a quite different appearance (Fig. 1.8, 1.9, 1.11), although based on the same data. An objection to this type of plot is that calculation of small ligand concentrations by extrapolation may be awkward, since the part of the scale covering these concentrations is cramped. However, an arithmetic scale may offer practical advantages if the assay is directed to a relatively narrow range of values (Fig. 1.15, an enlarged portion of Fig. 1.8). It also permits plotting of the zero standard as a point on the horizontal axis which is not possible with a logarithmic plot.

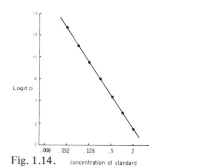

Fig. 1.14.

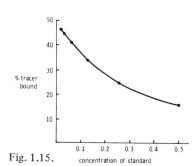

Fig. 1.15.

Fig. 1.8 – 1.15. The standard curve of Fig. 1.3 is plotted in various ways. Superficially the appearances are very different although based on identical data.

1.7.   The measurement of K value

The K value for any system can be calculated from the data contained in a standard curve, redrawn according to the method of Scatchard. Assuming that the binder is homogeneous and has a single K value, the 'Scatchard plot', with the bound/free ratio on the vertical axis and the bound fraction on the horizontal axis, yields a straight line, the slope of which is equal to the K value, and the intercept of which on the horizontal axis gives the absolute concentration of binder (Fig. 1.16). The basis of this relationship can be explained by further consideration of eq. (1.4):

$$\frac{[\text{AgAb}]}{[\text{Ag}][\text{Ab}]} = K \tag{1.4}$$

For the sake of simplicity, substitute X for [AgAb], the concentration of the bound complex at equilibrium; use Ag to describe the total concentrations of antigen in the system, and Ab to describe the total concentration of antibody. Equation (1.3) then becomes:

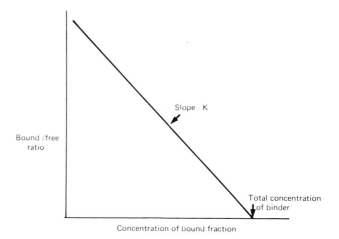

Fig. 1.16. Diagram of a Scatchard plot. For a system with a single affinity constant (K value) this yields a straight line of slope $-K$ which intercepts the horizontal axis at a value equivalent to the total concentration of the binder.

$$\frac{X}{(Ag - X)(Ab - X)} = K \tag{1.9}$$

Multiplying both sides by (Ab − X) gives us:

$$\frac{X}{(Ag - X)} = K(Ab - X) \tag{1.10}$$

or

$$\frac{X}{(Ag - X)} = K \cdot Ab - KX \tag{1.11}$$

Examining the equation in this form it can be seen that on the left-hand side X is equivalent to the bound fraction and (Ag − X) to the free. Therefore $X/(Ag - X)$, is the bound/free ratio. On the right-hand side both K and Ab are constants; so too is $K \cdot Ab$. The variable is $-KX$. Thus, a plot of $X/(Ag - X)$, the bound/free ratio, against X, the bound fraction, gives a straight line with slope $-K$. This is the Scatchard plot*.

The amount of antibody Ab, is given by the intercept on the horizontal axis, in other words, where the bound/free ratio is 0. Substituting in eq. (1.10):

$$0 = K \cdot Ab - KX \tag{1.12}$$

so

$$K \cdot Ab = KX \tag{1.13}$$

and

$$Ab = X \tag{1.14}$$

* A number of alternatives to the Scatchard plot have been described, including the Eisenthal and Cornish-Bowden plot (Eisenthal and Cornish-Bowden, 1974) and the Sips and Hill plot (Cornish-Bowden and Koshland, 1975). All use the same basic data and give effectively the same results.

Although simple in principle, in practice the measurement of K value can present many problems. This is particularly the case with antibodies. The apparent K value may vary with the concentration of the binder. Furthermore, with few exceptions most antisera to a given antigen will contain several populations of antibodies, each one with a different K value. Under these circumstances, the Scatchard plot is not a straight line, but instead a curve which represents a combination of the lines from each specific antibody population. The fact that antibody molecules are divalent, and that binding at one site may influence binding at the other should also be taken into account, as well as the possibility that the separation system disrupts the equilibrium. Another type of problem is seen with the naturally occurring binding proteins, such as cortisol-binding globulin; the apparent K value varies according to the temperature at which it is measured, being greater at $4°C$ than at $37°C$. A similar but less striking variation may be seen with antibodies to peptides, whereas antibodies to steroids or other small haptens show little or no variation (Keane et al., 1976).

K values of antibodies in commonly used radioimmunoassays range from $10^9 - 10^{12}$ l/mol. As a very approximate rule of thumb, the sensitivity is equivalent to $1/K$; thus the detection range will extend to 10^{-12} mol/l, or 1 pmol/l.

1.8. A model system for binding assays

If a reasonable estimate of K value can be made this can be used to predict the characteristics of the assay at various concentrations of reagents. A simple model will be described here, derived from the Law of Mass Action, which can be readily adapted to a programmable calculator. The principle is to take eq. (9):

$$\frac{X}{(Ag - X)(Ab - X)} = K \qquad (1.9)$$

and to turn it into quadratic form so that it can be rapidly solved for any set of values entered:

$$[Ag][Ab] - X[Ab] + (1/K) + X^2 = 0 \qquad (1.15)$$

A solution in terms of percentage is provided by the equation:

$$\text{Percent bound} = (a - \sqrt{a^2 - b})\, c \qquad (1.16)$$

where $a = [Ab] + [Ag] + 1/K$; $b = 4[Ag][Ab]$; $c = 50/[Ag]$.

1.9. An application of the model system

The model system can be used to determine the optimal concentration of tracer for use in an assay (see § 9.2.1). A series of binder dilution curves using successively smaller concentrations of tracer yields the pattern shown in Fig. 1.17 for both the model system and a real system. Reduction of tracer concentration leads to a shift of the curve to the right and the concentration of binder required to bind 50% of the tracer progressively

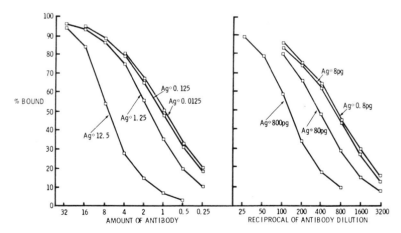

Fig. 1.17. Antibody dilution curves derived from a theoretical model of a radio-immunoassay (left) and from a radioimmunoassay for oxytocin (right). Ag* represents labelled antigen. Note that in both systems there is a limiting concentration of tracer antigen below which there is no further shift in the position of the dilution curve.

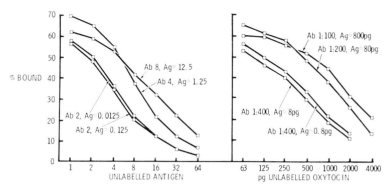

Fig. 1.18. Standard curves derived from a theoretical model of a radioimmunoassay (left) and from a radioimmunoassay for oxytocin (right). Ag* represents labelled antigen. Note that in both systems there is a limiting concentration of tracer antigen below which there is no further shift in the position of the standard curve.

decreases. However, beyond a certain point, further reduction produces no significant shift of the curve or of apparent titre. The point at which this occurs is determined entirely by the K value of the binder with respect to the ligand, and the limiting level of tracer in a series of binder dilution curves is also the limiting level for use in a standard curve. This is illustrated in Fig. 1.18. Reduction of tracer concentration in a series of standard curves results in a progressive shift to the left and an increase in the sensitivity of the system. But at the same limiting concentration of tracer seen in the dilution curves, there is no further change in the standard curves.

Thus, given a single standard curve in well-defined conditions it is possible to estimate the K value and to use this in the model system to evaluate different reagent concentrations. The results would have to be checked experimentally, but the procedure could eliminate a considerable amount of trial and error and provide a better understanding of the underlying basis of the technique. Equally, there are many systems in which the heterogeneity of the binder and the difficulty of estimating a single K value, would vitiate any simple attempt at theoretical analysis. Mathematical models which take into account the potential heterogeneity of binder-ligand systems have been described but are beyond the scope of this book (e.g., Feldman et al., 1972).

CHAPTER 2

Requirements for binding assays – purified ligand

2.1. Requirements for a binding assay

The requirements for a binding assay are purified ligand, tracer ligand, a specific binder, a method for distinguishing bound and free ligand and, in some cases, a procedure for extracting the ligand from biological fluids.

2.2. The need for purified ligand

A supply of highly purified ligand is essential to the development of any binding assay. If highly purified material is freely available (e.g., many of the steroid hormones and synthetic small peptide hormones), then it will be routinely used for standardisation, for preparation of tracer, for immunisation, and for monitoring recovery from biological fluids. If appropriate material is in very short supply (e.g., some substances from biological sources), relatively less pure material may be used at some stages of the system. But this is a compromise, and at some point at least one of the basic reagents must be pure.

2.3. Availability of pure ligand

It is impossible to discuss here all the ligands currently in use in binding assays. Instead, examples will be considered which illustrate some of the problems which may arise. A single generalisation may, however, be made: that ligands prepared synthetically (e.g., steroids, small peptide hormones, drugs) present relatively few problems, while ligands which have to be prepared from natural sources (e.g., large protein hormones, carcino-fetal antigens) can present considerable problems. As with all generalisations, exceptions will be encountered.

2.3.1. Large protein hormones

The first radioimmunoassays, for insulin, suffered problems due to the difficulty in obtaining adequate supplies of pure hormone of human origin. These problems no longer exist, since supplies of both synthetic and highly purified natural material are available.

Similar problems have arisen with the various hormones of the anterior pituitary gland, particularly the glycoproteins, LH, FSH and TSH. Preparations of these are available from international agencies but their purity, as judged by biological potency per unit weight, is invariably less than that of the most highly purified preparations reported by individual workers. Furthermore, the most widely used preparations of the gonadotrophins were derived from post-menopausal urine and intended for use in bioassay*; from the immunochemical point of view these differ significantly from the corresponding hormone in both the pituitary and the circulation. Standards are also available which consist of purified pituitary material**, but none are identical to each other, or to circulating endogenous LH and FSH (Rosemberg, 1979; Storring et al., 1981; Zaida et al., 1982).

2.3.2. Carcino-fetal antigens

The best known of these are alpha-fetoprotein (AFP) and carcinoembryonic antigen (CEA). Highly purified AFP is now fairly easily obtained; it is abundant in the tissue of origin (fetal serum, fetal liver), and fetal material is, in many countries, readily available. Although CEA is also abundant in the tissue of origin (colo-rectal carcinomas), the purified materials are less satisfactory because they exhibit the heterogeneity

---

* 2nd International Reference Preparation of human menopausal gonadotrophin (1964); 1st International Standard for urinary FSH and urinary hLH (1976)
** WHO Reference Preparation 69/104 for hFSH and hLH (also known as LER 907); 1st International Reference Preparation of human pituitary LH for immunoassay, MRC 68/40

which seems to be characteristic of all glycoproteins prepared from natural sources. This heterogeneity, and the resulting possibility of cross-reaction with normally occurring antigens, may explain why the measurement of circulating CEA as an index of malignancy is less specific than was originally thought to be the case. It must also explain why no two systems of CEA assay give identical results, even using identical standards (Sizaret and Esteve, 1980).

2.3.3. Steroid hormones, drugs and other small molecules

Since the majority of these compounds are prepared chemically, material of virtually 100% purity is usually available in good quantities from commercial sources. However, purity should not always be assumed, and it is essential for any laboratory setting up a new assay to check their basic materials (e.g., by thin-layer or gas–liquid chromatography and mass spectroscopy). Furthermore, problems may arise because of instability of the material. For example, the predominant form of folate in serum samples is N^5-methyltetrahydrofolic acid (N^5-MTHF). Since this is unstable unless kept at low temperature, many workers have chosen to use pteroylglutamic acid (PGA) for standardisation (Givas and Gutcho, 1975). At pH 9.5 PGA and N^5-MTHF have similar affinity for folate binding proteins.

2.3.4. Small peptide hormones

The most familiar of these (e.g., oxytocin, arginine vasopressin, angiotensin, LH/FSH releasing hormone, TSH releasing hormone) are prepared synthetically to a high degree of purity. For the laboratory which cannot do this for itself (i.e., the majority) availability usually depends on pharmaceutical interest in this material. Thus synthetic oxytocin, which is widely used in the induction of labour, is freely available in milligram quantities. By contrast, arginine-vasopressin (AVP), which is the naturally occurring antidiuretic hormone of most mammalian species, is relatively difficult to obtain because the analogue prepared for clinical use is lysine-vasopressin (LVP).

As with steroids and drugs, it should not be assumed that synthetic peptides are invariably 100% pure. In the course of preparation 'error' peptides are likely to be produced and free amino acids to remain. Furthermore, alterations may occur with storage, in particular oxidation and the formation of dimers. All such preparations should be examined both physicochemically (e.g., by thin-layer chromatography) and by biological assay before they are used in any other assay system.

2.4. Dissimilarity between purified ligand and endogenous ligand

Ideally the ligand used in an assay (as tracer and standard) should be identical with the endogenous ligand which that assay is intended to measure. Frequently this is not the case; there are many examples of such dissimilarities, including:

(1) *Species differences*: The use of animal materials in radioimmunoassays for human hormones has been very common in the past; for instance, material of bovine origin in assays for insulin and for parathormone.

(2) *Strain differences*: Hepatitis B antigen occurs in various types; a common determinant designated '*a*', and one from each of two pairs of mutually exclusive determinants '*d*', '*y*', and '*w*', '*r*' (Le Bouvier, 1972).

(3) *Tissue differences*: The exact tissue or fluid of origin can be very critical. Glucagon prepared from gut differs immunochemically from pancreatic glucagon (Bloom, 1974). The peptides released by 'ACTH-secreting' tumours may be very different from normal pituitary ACTH (Rees, 1976). The immunochemical nature of the glycoprotein hormones (LH, FSH, TSH) differs according to whether they are prepared from urine or pituitary extracts (see Franchimont, 1971). Growth hormone (GH) exists in a multiplicity of different forms in the pituitary and blood. These forms have different biological activities, and widely differing potencies in immunoassays (Vodian and Nicoll, 1979; Sigel et al. 1980). This may explain why bioassays of plasma GH can give much higher results than those of radioimmunoassay.

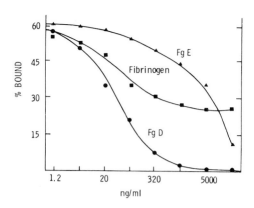

Fig. 2.1. Standard curves for fibrinogen and its degradation products fragment D (FgD) and E (FgE) using ^{125}I-labelled FgD as tracer and an antiserum to FgD. Note that fibrinogen shows only partial cross-reaction in this assay although it must, by definition, contain the sequences which make up FgD. (From data kindly supplied by Dr. Y.B. Gordon.)

(4) *Multiple forms of the material*: There are many instances when the endogenous material may occur in several different forms. Insulin is synthesised as a single large precursor molecule, 'pro-insulin'; at the time of release this is broken down to yield the two peptide chains of authentic insulin, together with the connecting peptide chain or 'C-peptide' (Steiner et al., 1968). Under certain conditions pro-insulin is released into the circulation, but this will not be revealed by the majority of insulin assays. Metabolism of the endogenous material may also lead to non-identity. For example, fibrinogen cross-reacts only partly in a radioimmunoassay for the fibrinogen degradation product, FgD (Fig. 2.1) (Gordon et al., 1973). Metabolites of a hormone may give positive results in a radioimmunoassay for that hormone, and thus provide a poor reflection of the biological activity (see § 12.4). Conjugates of steroids react poorly or not at all with antisera to the non-conjugated molecule and in most cases would not be detected in an assay directed to the latter.

2.5. Standards

Differences between laboratories in reagents and protocol for a given assay will inevitably yield a wide range of different results for the same material. In order to overcome this problem, considerable efforts have been directed towards the use by all groups of a single material as standard. The preparation and distribution of common standard materials of this type has now become a function of the World Health Organisation, the principle agencies being the National Institute for Biological Standards and Control of the Medical Research Council in the United Kingdom, and the National Pituitary Agency of the National Institute of Arthritis, Metabolism and Digestive Diseases in the USA.

2.5.1. Characteristics of a standard

The purpose of standardisation by the use of common reference materials is to permit expression of results which are consistent between different laboratories, and at different times in the same laboratory. A material intended as a standard should have certain characteristics (Bangham and Cotes, 1974):

(1) It should be available in quantities large enough to supply many laboratories for many years;

(2) It should be stable, and the effects of storage for several months at different temperatures should be carefully examined;

(3) It should not contain substances which can interefere with assays, and for this reason it must be tested in a wide variety of assay systems before it is distributed;

(4) Ideally it should contain highly purified substance (i.e., a single molecular species) but this is sometimes impossible for the reasons already discussed under the heading of availability.

2.5.2. Preparation and calibration of an international standard

The usual procedure for setting up a standard is to obtain a large quantity of the relevant material, and then to aliquot it as identical volumes of a solution into several hundred neutral glass ampoules. These are then stored at low temperature. Alternatively, the ampoules are freeze-dried as a single batch and then sealed under nitrogen. This is particularly convenient because it permits distribution through ordinary postal services; by contrast, material in solution should be maintained in the frozen state until it is used. The disadvantage of freeze-drying is that it may produce considerable alterations in a molecule.

Once a new international standard has been prepared it is calibrated against previous standards by assay in several expert laboratories and the averaged results form the basis for assignment of a unitage to the new standard. In cases in which there is disagreement among the expert groups, the estimation of the mean can become statistically very complex.

2.5.3. Practical use of standards

As a general rule, when a widely available standard is used to calibrate an assay system, the result should be expressed in terms of that standard, and not arbitrarily converted to other units. This rule is often broken. For example, the international reference preparations for human LH (e.g., MRC 68/40) are distributed in ampoules whose contents are defined in Units; this is necessary because the contained material has not been fully characterised by physicochemical means. It is not uncommon for workers to convert the results obtained using this standard to an absolute estimate of weight, using a conversion factor based on the biological activity per unit weight of highly purified LH. There are three drawbacks to this procedure:

(1) It is always unwise to extrapolate from an assay based on structure to an assay based on function;
(2) The biological activity of the standard is disputed, since different assay systems give different results;
(3) The biological activity of available preparations of highly purified LH is also disputed.

Thus, conversion to weight gives a spurious impression of accuracy which is not justified by the basic facts.

Many laboratories conducting binding assays on a large scale use their own materials as working standards, and calibrate these from time to time against the appropriate international standards. This is also a universal practice in the manufacture of radioimmunoassay kits, since materials from the World Health Organisation are not available for commercial distribution. No exception can be taken to the use of working standards provided that calibration is adequately carried out, and that it is always appreciated that the material is not necessarily identical with the international standard. It may, for example, be inferior in terms of stability, a fact which can pass unrecognised unless stringent tests are carried out. On the other hand, it is quite possible for a working standard to be superior to the international standard, especially in terms of physicochemical homogeneity. Thus, it would be impossible to explore the specificity of radioimmunoassay for oxytocin and vasopressin using the international standard for these hormones which contains a mixture of the two. Problems may also arise when a working standard yields a dose-response curve which is non-parallel to the international standard, thus making quantitative comparison difficult or impossible. This is the situation encountered when assays for circulating LH based on highly purified pituitary LH are compared with an international standard (the 2nd IRP/HMG) consisting of hormone extracted from urine.

Finally, it should be emphasised that the existence of an international reference material may help towards, but cannot guarantee, homogeneity of results between different laboratories. The specificity of other reagents used in the assay is of equal importance (see Ch. 9 and § 2.3.2). This applies even if the reference material itself is absolutely pure (which is rarely the case).

The preparation of standards is possibly the single most important step in ensuring the clinical efficiency of an assay. Some practical recommendations for the preparation of standards are shown in Table 2.1. In some cases 'ligand'-free serum is necessary as a medium (e.g., thyroxine) and a typical protocol for this is shown in Table 2.2.

TABLE 2.1

Preparation of standards (see Das, 1980)

This should invariably be carried out by skilled and reliable personnel, using the best available balances and volumetric glassware.

Standards should be prepared as individual dilutions from a master standard and a scheme for this is set out below, taking human placental lactogen as an example:

1. Weigh out 10 mg highly purified hPL (ILS Ltd).
2. Dissolve in 10 ml hPL-free serum (from a non-pregnant human or an animal species).
3. Dispense as aliquots of 0.5 ml and store deep-frozen in closed tubes.
4. Dilute an aliquot 1 : 10 (0.4 ml + 3.6 ml hPL-free serum) to give a solution of 100 μg/ml.
5. Set out 6 tubes each containing 10 ml of hPL-free serum.
6. Remove an appropriate volume from each tube and replace it with the solution from (4) above:

Tube no.	Volume exchanged (ml)	Standard concentration (μg/ml)
1	1.2	12
2	0.8	8
3	0.6	6
4	0.4	4
5	0.2	2
6	0.1	1

Deep-freeze as aliquots each sufficient for 1 week of assays (0.2–0.4 ml)

Note: The largest available amount of standard is weighed out to ensure maximum accuracy and precision assuming use of a microgram balance. When International standards or reference preparations are supplied they are usually accompanied by instructions similar to steps 1 and 2

2.5.3.1. Rules for preparation of standards

(1) Individual sets of standards should always be prepared as aliquots from a larger pool made at each concentration.

(2) Each standard concentration should be prepared independently from a solution of master standard. The use of doubling dilutions is much to be deprecated because it can lead to cumulative errors (Fig. 2.2).

TABLE 2.2

Preparation of ligand-free sera for standards

For many naturally occurring materials which are not species-specific a source of ligand-free serum may not be readily available. In the case of small molecules such as cortisol and thyroxine it is possible to prepare ligand-free serum by treatment with a potent adsorbent such as charcoal. All steps should be carried out in the cold

1. Add 10 g of dry, unwashed Norit OL charcoal to 100 ml plasma or serum.
2. Mix overnight on a magnetic stirrer or by vertical rotation.
3. Centrifuge for 1 h at 10,000 x g or higher to remove the bulk of the charcoal.
4. Pass through a sequence of Millipore filters (e.g., 7, 5, 2 and 0.22 μm) to remove remaining charcoal.

The efficiency of the extraction can be monitored by the addition of a small amount of labelled material (e.g., ^{125}I-labelled thyroxine). It is important that all the charcoal should be removed since even trace amounts can interfere with the assay.

Note: Removal of vitamin B12 from serum by charcoal is very inefficient. An alternative method is treatment with ascorbate and dialysis

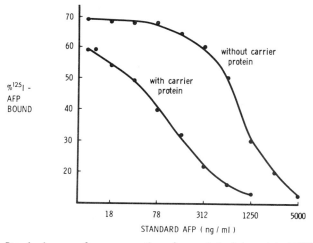

Fig. 2.2. Standard curves for a preparation of pure alpha-fetoprotein (AFP) serially diluted in the presence and absence of carrier protein (2 mg/ml bovine serum albumin). With no protein there is a progressive loss due to absorption to the tube and incomplete transfer leading to gross non-parallelism. (From data kindly supplied by Dr. M. Al-Awqati.)

(3) Standards should always be prepared in the largest possible batches, assuming that the material is stable on storage. Because every step of sampling and dispensing has an error, no two sets of standards prepared on different occasions from the same primary materials can ever be identical. Frequent changes of standards will inevitably lead to an increase in the long-term assay coefficient of variation (see Ch. 11), and may also be associated with a persistent 'drift' of quality control values. The aim should be to prepare sufficient sets of assay standards to last for at least 1 year and preferably longer. These batches should, in turn, be prepared from a 'master standard' – a single solution of concentrated standard which is prepared with great care and aliquoted to yield sufficient material for several years' operation of an assay. Sometimes this is impractical, for example if insufficient material is available, or if one standard preparation is replaced by another.

(4) The stability of standards may be improved by freeze-drying. However, this introduces additional sources of error since both the initial dispensing and the reconstitution must be quantitative. Liquid or deep-frozen standards (§ 2.6) avoid both these steps, the only error being in the final dispensing into the assay tube.

(5) Standards should always be prepared in solutions containing a bulk protein (e.g., albumin, whole serum) because of the inherent instability of many biological materials in very dilute solutions.

It is difficult to make general recommendations with respect to the 'spacing' of standards which is often a technically convenient mathematical progression but may be unrelated to the logic of the assay. However, three general comments can be made:

(1) Standards should not be chosen in such a manner that the experimental difference between successive points is very small (for most common assays the binding difference should be at least 4–5%;

(2) It is good practice to choose as one standard a concentration value which is considered to represent the cut-off between normality and abnormality (e.g., 2.5 ng/ml in a digoxin assay);

(3) The standard defined in (2) above should never lie at either extreme of the standard curve.

2.6. *Storage of materials used in binding assays*

This is an appropriate place to consider some aspects of reagent storage, whether standard, binder, tracer, or samples for assay. The number of possible materials is vast ranging from those, such as aqueous solutions of drugs, which are stable almost indefinitely at room temperature, to others such as small peptides in plasma, which may be destroyed in a matter of hours. However, certain generalisations may be made. Most biological materials are more stable at low temperature, and it is usual to store them in the frozen state. Three specific points should be made about the freezing of solutions of biological materials:

(1) The freezing point of whole serum is probably around $-22°C$ and the process of freezing can be very damaging unless carried out rapidly; in normal domestic freezers the process is slow, and can easily lead to damage due to formation of large ice crystals*; initial freezing in liquid nitrogen or a mixture of dry ice and ethanol, is much more rapid and satisfactory.

(2) The rate of initial cooling is probably as important as the eventual temperature at which the material is kept.

(3) Repeated cycles of freezing and thawing are highly detrimental to the majority of biological molecules. If a given material has to be removed frequently from a deep freeze, then it should be stored in aliquots small enough to obviate the need for re-freezing.

---

* As a solution cooled ice crystals of pure water will form which exclude solute molecules. Eventually the latter reach a critical concentration (the 'eutectic concentration') at which the mixture freezes solid. The formation of ice crystals leaves pockets of concentrated solute; proteins in these pockets can be damaged by the high salt concentrations until the whole mixture is frozen

Another aspect of storage is the chemical environment of the material. Proteins should always be kept at a concentration of 1 mg/ml or greater; a diluted antiserum loses activity much more rapidly than the corresponding neat antiserum. If the material is not available at sufficiently high concentration, then the addition of a carrier protein (Table 1.5) should be considered. Some biological molecules such as ACTH are particularly liable to damage by oxidation, and may be better stored in the presence of a reducing agent, or in an oxygen-free atmosphere. Other factors include the pH and ionic strength of the environment.

Stability can often be enhanced by freeze-drying and storage in a heat-sealed ampoule or rubber-stoppered vial under an atmosphere of dry nitrogen*. With some purified proteins in aqueous solutions the freeze-drying process may lead to formation of aggregates; this is unlikely to affect standards prepared in whole serum, or tracer or antibody prepared in buffers containing carrier proteins such as serum albumin (Table 1.5). If part of the material is to be kept in powder form after the ampoule is opened it should be stored in the dark in an evacuated desiccator or in a sealed polythene bag containing silica gel. All materials should be kept in a refrigerator or deep-freeze when not in use.

---

* The half-life of biological activity of the International Standard for corticotrophin under these conditions has been estimated at 2800 years! (Storring et al., 1980)

CHAPTER 3

Requirements for binding assays – tracer ligand using radioisotopic labels

Essential to any binding assay is a means for determining the distribution between the bound and free fractions. For this purpose, a small amount of highly purified labelled ligand (the 'tracer') is incorporated in the system. The label may be any substance having the primary characteristic that it can be measured accurately by direct and simple methods, and that the sensitivity with which it can be detected is greater than that of direct methods for the measurement of the ligand itself. The most commonly used label is a radioactive isotope. Other labels, such as enzymes and fluorescent molecules which meet the criteria described above, can equally be used and are described in detail in the next chapter.

This chapter will begin with a short account of radioactive isotopes and their detection, and continue with a description of the characteristics and preparation of tracers intended for use in a binding assay.

3.1. Radioactive isotopes

An atom of any element consists of a central nucleus around which rotate electrons. The nucleus contains two main types of particle, protons and neutrons; these are of approximately the same mass, but the protons carry a positive electrical charge, while the neutrons are uncharged. Electrons carry a negative electrical charge equal to that of the proton, but their mass is only 1/1840 of that of a proton; for this reason, the mass of an atom is roughly the same as the total mass of protons and neutrons in the nucleus. The number of protons, or 'atomic number' determines the chemical characteristics of an atom and defines its position as an element in the periodic table. With many elements, the number of neutrons in the nucleus is variable, leading to differences in atomic mass but not in chemical properties. The term 'isotope' is applied to these variants. Hydrogen, for example, can exist in three isotopic forms; in the simplest and commonest, there is a single proton in the nucleus and one electron in an orbital ring. Less common are forms in which the mass is increased by the addition of one or two neutrons, referred to as 'deuterium' and 'tritium', respectively. Individual isotopes are referred to by the symbol for the element with the atomic mass written as a superscript, e.g., ^{1}H, ^{2}H, ^{3}H; the atomic number (number of protons) is sometimes included as a subscript, e.g., $^1_1$H, $^2_1$H, $^3_1$H.

The nucleus of some isotopes is unstable, and these are known as 'radioactive isotopes'. Under these circumstances the nucleus will undergo spontaneous transformation to a more stable state, and in the process will emit energy in the form of either particles or non-particulate electromagnetic vibrations such as γ-rays, or X-rays. The following processes may be involved:

(1) Expulsion of an α-particle (2 protons and 2 neutrons, equivalent to a helium nucleus). This occurs only with heavy elements.

(2) Conversion of a neutron into a proton, an electron, and a neutrino (a small uncharged particle); the last two are expelled (β-emission).

(3) Conversion of a proton into a neutron, a positron (a positively charged electron), and a neutrino; the last two are expelled (β-emission).

(4) Electron capture, in which a nuclear proton is converted to a neutron by the capture of an orbital electron; the process leads to emission of weak X-rays.

(5) Isomeric transition, in which an unstable nucleus changes to a more stable isomer, the excess energy being emitted as γ-rays.

(6) Internal conversion of γ-rays leading to emission of an orbital electron.

As a result of the first three of these processes the nucleus will have a different atomic number, but the atomic mass may be the same or lower. If the residual conformation of the nucleus is still unstable, further transformations occur until it becomes stable.

The rate of disintegration (or 'decay') of a given radioactive isotope is specific to that isotope; it is described by the 'half-life', the time required for 50% of the radioisotope to decay. The unit of radioactivity, originally defined as the radioactivity of 1 g radium, is the 'Curie' where:

1 Curie (Ci)= 3.7×10^{10} dps
1 milliCurie (mCi) = 3.7×10^{7} dps
1 microCurie (μCi) = 3.7×10^{4} dps

In the new 'Système Internationale' the unit of radioactivity is the bequerel (bq) which is 1 dps. Typical conversion factors are:

1 Curie (Ci) = 37 gigabequerels (GBq)
1 milliCurie (mCi) = 37 megabequerels (MBq)
1 microCurie (μCi) = 37 kilobequerels (kBq)

The radioactivity of a sample of an isotope will thus depend on the amount of isotope present, and its half-life.

3.2. Counting of radioactive isotopes

Detection and quantitation of an isotope in a radioimmunoassay depends on the use of a scintillation counter; the essential parts of this system are a scintillator, a photomultiplier tube and electronic circuits (Fig. 3.1).

A scintillator is a material which emits a light flash when struck by ionising radiation; the intensity of the flash varies with the energy of the radiation. The light flashes are detected by a photomultiplier, which converts them into electrical pulses. The amplitude of these pulses is proportional to the intensity of the scintillation, and thus to the energy of the radiation which produced it. For any given isotope the radiation shows a continuous distribution of energies, or spectrum, with a maximum which is characteristic of that isotope. By means of pulse-height analysis a scintillation counter can be set to detect pulses with a narrow range of amplitude, and thus to count an isotope with minimal interference from other isotopes or background radiation (Fig. 3.2).

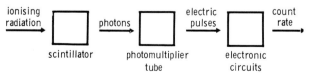

Fig. 3.1. The principle of scintillation counting.

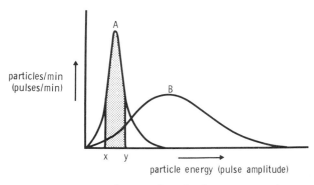

Fig. 3.2. The energy spectra of two radioactive isotopes, A and B. By setting a 'window' on the counter which sees only energies lying between *x* and *y* most of the radiation from isotope A will be counted, but little of that from isotope B.

The type of scintillator used depends on the nature of the radiation emitted, which in practical terms means either β-particles (from isotopes such as ^{3}H or ^{14}C) or γ-rays (from isotopes such as ^{131}I or ^{125}I). Beta particles have very low penetrating power in matter, and can only be detected when the isotope is in intimate contact with the scintillator. For this purpose, a solution in an aromatic solvent is made of the isotope together with an aromatic compound which has the property of fluorescing (i.e., emitting light) when excited by ionising radiation. The most widely used compound is 2,5-diphenyloxazole (PPO). Aqueous solutions may be relatively insoluble in aromatic solvents such as toluene and xylene. To overcome this, the scintillation 'cocktail' includes a non-ionic detergent such as Triton X-100; an appropriate mixture of this type can accept up to 30% (v/v) of an aqueous sample. The efficiency of a liquid scintillator can be much reduced by the presence of impurities such as proteins; this is the phenomenon known as 'quenching', and corrections may be necessary if the solutions counted differ widely in composition (e.g. standards prepared in simple buffer while the unknowns are samples of whole plasma). Liquid scintillation counting is discussed in detail by Fox, in Vol. 5/I of this series.

In contrast to β-particles, γ-rays have high penetrating power. Intimate contact between the isotope and the scintillator is therefore unnecessary, and the scintillator consists of a crystal of sodium iodide coated with thallium, usually formed as a well; as the radiation strikes the molecules making up the crystal lattice, ionisation occurs and results in a light flash which is then detected by the photomultiplier. Because some γ-rays may be partially quenched by glass, the use of plastic tubes is always recommended.

Gamma-counting is much simpler and cheaper than liquid scintillation counting. No sample preparation is required, giving considerable savings in time and materials. The specific activities of γ-emitting isotopes are much greater than those of β-emitters, so that counting times are reduced or alternatively, smaller amounts of tracer can be counted in the same time. These characteristics are summarised in Table 3.1.

3.3. Choice of counter*

A wide variety of equipment is available for both liquid and crystal scintillation counting. For a given technical specification there is little to choose between the products of different manufacturers, and the final decision is likely to rest with factors such as cost and availability of service; the latter is particularly critical for users who work at any distance from major cities. The following specific factors should be taken into account:

TABLE 3.1
Comparison of the characteristics of a commonly used γ-emitting isotope (^{125}I) with that of β-emitters (^{14}C and ^{3}H)

Isotope	Half-life	Atoms/Ci	Detection efficiency (%)	No. of atoms equivalent to 1 detectable atom of ^{125}I
^{125}I	60 days	2.77×10^{17}	80	1
^{14}C	5730 years	9.65×10^{21}	85	37,010
^{3}H	12.26 years	2.08×10^{19}	55	51.6

* An excellent and detailed review of the principles and choice of a γ-counter is available (Wilde and Ottewell, 1980)

(1) *Liquid or crystal scintillation counter*:   This is determined by the intended application. The much greater convenience of γ-counting means that whenever possible a γ-emitting isotope is used, and β-emitters are used only when there is no alternative. Until quite recently the latter applied to most small molecules (e.g., steroid hormones); increasingly, however, γ-labelled tracers are becoming available for all materials of biomedical interest, and the day is foreseeable when liquid scintillation counting will be little used in the context of routine assays.

(2) *Manual or automatic sampling changing*:   This is determined by a balance between requirements and finance. If the total counting time required is less than 1 h/day (e.g., 60 tubes counted for 1 min each) then an automatic changer is unnecessary. For larger throughputs an automatic changer is essential; although the capital cost is at least 5 times that of a manual model, the savings in technician time and the ability to operate for 24 h a day will more than repay the extra cost.

(3) *Sample capacity*:   For an automatic system, this should be in the range 100–500. Equipment of larger capacity is cumbersome, a id only of value if counting times are very short. A point of considerable practical importance is the transit time between samples (i.e., the time taken between the ending of counts on one tube and the beginning of counts on the next). For efficient operation this should be as short as possible as it can make a large difference to total counting time (e.g., 10 sec counts of 500 tubes with a transit time of 30 sec will take 5.5 h; with a transit time of 10 sec the total time is less than 3 h).

(4) *Size of crystal*:   Most γ-counters have a well-type crystal 2 in. or 3 in. diameter. Although the crystal may be more efficient for emitters of high penetration, it is expensive and liable to yield high background values. For most purposes, and certainly for ^{125}I which is the most commonly used isotope, the larger crystal is unnecessary.

(5) *Single or multiple detectors*:   Gamma-counting equipment is now available with multiple detector heads (e.g., Nuclear Enterprises NE1600; Innotron 'Hydragamma'). Several samples can be counted simultaneously, representing a considerable saving in time, space, and money for users

with a high throughput. With the introduction of microprocessor control and batch processing techniques, these are almost certainly the systems of the future.

(6) *Electronic circuits and controls*: In the context of assay work, these should be as simple as possible. The great complexity of some equipment, particularly that intended for liquid scintillation counting and designed to permit simultaneous measurement of a mixture of isotopes in several different channels, is usually quite unnecessary. For most purposes a single channel machine is adequate and cost-saving. Furthermore, several recent models are '^{125}I-dedicated', in other words, set to count only this commonly used isotope; the addition of a channel to count ^{57}Co, for vitamin B12 assays, might well become redundant in the light of the recent development of a ^{125}I-labelled B12 tracer (Endres et al., 1978). The only control in which versatility is essential is the count timer, which should be adjustable in steps of 1 sec over $1 - \geqslant 1000$ sec.

(7) *Output*: All types of counter usually incorporate a digital scalar. For automatic changers, an output printer is also necessary. More sophisticated equipment sometimes incorporates a 'micro-computer', capable of data reduction and on-line analysis of results (see § 8.6). With the introduction of relatively inexpensive systems this is now highly desirable, particularly with multiple detector counters.

3.4. Some practical aspects of isotope counting

(1) *Choice of counting time*: The error of a count is approximately proportional to the square root of the total number of counts accumulated: for 1000 counts the error is 10, or 10%, for 10,000 counts the error is 100 or 1%. All tubes of an assay should be counted for sufficient time to yield total counts with an error not greater than that introduced by other steps in the assay procedure. For practical purposes, the minimum number of counts accumulated for any tube should be 2000, with an error of approximately 2%. Accumulation of more than 10,000 counts is usually unnecessary and leads to an undesirable increase in counting time.

(2) *Fixed time or fixed total counts*: Many counters have the facility to accumulate a fixed number of counts and to present the result as a variable of time. This has the advantage that the counting error for all tubes is identical but for tubes containing low levels of activity counting times may be very prolonged. A new development is the use of an on-line microprocessor which automatically adjusts counting time so that the error of the counts is roughly equivalent to the experimental error for a given point – in other words, counting proceeeds only for so long as is statistically useful (Ekins et al., 1978).

(3) *Background counts and background subtraction*: A well-maintained γ-counter with adequate shielding around the crystal should not yield more than 50 cpm as background. This can usually be ignored, and background subtraction is unnecessary. High background counts (100 cpm or more) may arise for several reasons:

(*i*) Mis-setting of electronic controls;
(*ii*) Contamination of the crystal with isotope;
(*iii*) Contamination of a carrier or an automatic sample changer;
(*iv*) Presence of a powerful radioactive source near the crystal.

Means for the correction of these are obvious. The major problem arises with contamination of a crystal; repeated washing with detergent and ethanol may be necessary, and unless carried out with great care the thallium coating can be damaged. With liquid scintillation counting, background subtraction is widely used; the low specific activity of β-emitters imposes long counting times, and under these circumstances background counts may form a substantial proportion of the total.

(4) *For γ-counting of precipitates, liquids, sections of paper strips, etc.*: Any type of plastic tube which will fit the well of the crystal can be used. Counting can be performed without any further preparation of the sample. If the volume or size of the sample is such that some extends above the opening of the well then some counting efficiency may be lost. Given a choice between counting the bound fraction or counting the free fraction (e.g., between the precipitate and the supernatant with most separation procedures), it is a general rule to count the smaller of the two fractions which is usually the bound.

Manufacturers of counting equipment are shown in Appendix I.

3.5. Essential characteristics of a tracer

Since the tracer is intended simply to provide a measure of the total ligand in the bound and free phases of the system, it is obvious that its behaviour must be as nearly identical as possible with that of the unlabelled ligand. 'Behaviour', in this context, refers to its property of combination with the binder. Other properties may be a useful practical guide, but do not necessarily reflect what will happen in an assay system. For example, the labelling of a hapten or a small peptide may substantially alter its physicochemical properties, yet the behaviour in a binding assay may be virtually identical with that of unlabelled ligand. At the same time, small variations in a ligand which would be barely detectable in most systems of physicochemical analysis may dramatically alter its properties in combination with an antibody (e.g., oxidation of the methionine residue in ACTH). There is only one ultimate criterion for the properties of a tracer — that it should behave similarly with the unlabelled ligand in *the assay system*.

By definition the tracer must be slightly different from the pure ligand. Differences may arise, as noted above, because of the sheer presence of the label on the molecule. More important in practical terms, differences may arise because of alterations in the molecule, or the introduction of impurities, in the course of preparation. The general term for variations in the tracer which alter its binding properties is 'damage'. Any tracer or fraction of the tracer which reacts with the binder with a lower affinity than that of the unlabelled ligand can be described as damaged, and the causes of this are discussed below (§ 3.7.4).

3.6. Preparation of tracers

Tracers can be divided into two types: those with an internal label and those with an external label. With an internal label, an existing atom in the ligand molecule is replaced by a radioactive isotope of that atom (e.g., ^{14}C for ^{12}C, ^{3}H for ^{1}H), and the tracer should be identical with the unlabelled ligand. With an external label, an atom or atoms of a radioactive isotope (e.g., ^{131}I, ^{125}I) are covalently linked to an existing atom on the ligand molecule. A tracer with an external label is, by definition, not identical with the unlabelled ligand though in practice its behaviour may not be distinguishable from the latter. Tracers with an internal label are commonly used in the case of small molecules such as steroid hormones or drugs. They are usually prepared on a commercial scale by one of four methods:

(1) *Neutron bombardment of the compound in an atomic pile*:   This is not commonly used because it is unselective (i.e., may alter many atoms of different isotopic forms), and is likely to disrupt the molecule.

(2) *Chemical synthesis*:   The molecule is synthesised from simpler molecules or elements, one or more of which is in the form of a radioactive isotope; for example, the synthesis of vasopressin from its component amino acids, using [^{3}H]tyrosine.

(3) *Biological synthesis*:   The molecule is synthesised by a biological system in vivo or in vitro, using isotopically labelled precursors (e.g., prostaglandin $F_2\alpha$ from tritiated arachidonic acid).

(4) *Exchange reactions (Wilzbach technique)*:   Material for labelling is distributed over the walls of a tube, then exposed to tritium (^{3}H) gas at room temperature for one week; the process can be enhanced by the use of microwaves. The material is separated from free tritium and damaged products are removed by crystallisation and chromatography. This procedure yields tracers of high specific activity (up to 100 mCi/g), but the labelling is not necessarily uniform, nor is it specific to any particular site in the molecule.

3.7. Iodinated tracers

Tracers with an external label are commonly used in the case of larger peptide and protein molecules, and increasingly with haptens such as steroids and drugs because of the high specific activities which can be achieved (e.g., 2000–4000 Ci/mmol for an iodinated steroid rather than 25–100 Ci/mmol with an internal ^{3}H label). Isotopes of iodine are almost universally employed at present, and their use will be described in some detail. Precautions to be observed in handling these isotopes are set out in Appendix V.

3.7.1. *Iodination methods*

Iodine can be substituted on to the aromatic sidechain of tyrosine residues with relative ease (Fig. 3.3) yielding a stable compound which, if the iodine is in the form of a radioactive isotope such as ^{131}I or ^{125}I, forms a highly efficient tracer. Iodine may also substitute on to other amino acids, including histidine and phenylalanine, although the rate of the latter reaction is some 30–80-times less than that for tyrosine. The exact nature and location of the substitution on to tyrosine varies with specific activity, the nature of the peptide molecule and the method of iodination. At low levels of specific activity ($\leqslant 1$ iodine atom/molecule) the majority of substitutions are single (i.e., mono-iodotyrosine); only at higher levels of activity is diiodotyrosine formed. In a given molecule, tyrosine residues may differ widely in their accessibility. For example: insulin has four tyrosines, in positions 14 and 19 on the A chain, and 16 and 26 on the B chain; the majority of the iodine substitutes at position

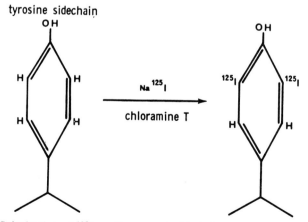

Fig. 3.3. Substitution of ^{125}I on the aromatic sidechain of tyrosine in the presence of the oxidising agent, chloramine T.

A14, some at A19, and very little at B16 or B26 (Freedlender and Cathou, 1971).

Many procedures have been described for iodination. The so-called 'direct' methods have in common the conversion of iodide (I^-), which is relatively unreactive, into a more reactive species such as free iodine (I_2), or positively charged iodine radicals (I^+), which can react with appropriate groups on the ligand. The basic chemistry of the reaction is poorly understood, the literature on the subject is conflicting, and will not be discussed further. The 'indirect' methods involve conjugation of ligand to a molecule already labelled with iodine (see below).

Methods of iodination are shown in Table 3.2.

3.7.1.1. Chloramine T (Greenwood et al., 1963)   Chloramine T, originally marketed as a disinfectant, is a potent oxidising agent capable of converting iodide to a more reactive form. The procedure is simple, requiring only mixing of solutions of the peptide, sodium iodide (^{125}I or ^{131}I), and chloramine T; the reaction is terminated by the addition of a reducing agent, sodium metabisulphite. The simplicity explains the wide acceptance of the technique and, as already noted, has done much to popularise the general application of radioimmunoassay. Practical aspects of the procedure are described in § 3.7.3 and Table 3.5.

TABLE 3.2
Iodination techniques

Technique	Authors
Iodine monochloride	McFarlane, 1958
Chloramine T*	Greenwood et al., 1963
Lactoperoxidase*	Marchalonis, 1969
Iodine vaporisation	Butt, 1972
Chlorine/hypochlorite	Redshaw and Lynch, 1974
Electrolysis	Rosa et al., 1979 and
	Nielsen et al., 1979
Conjugation labelling*	Bolton and Hunter, 1972
Iodogen*	Fraker and Speck, 1978

* Commonly used, see § 3.7.1.1 – 3.7.1.3

3.7.1.2. Lactoperoxidase (EC 1.11.1.7) (Marchalonis, 1969; Thorell and Johansson, 1971) Enzymatic iodination using lactoperoxidase in the presence of a trace of hydrogen peroxide has the advantage that the peptide is not exposed to high concentrations of a chemical oxidising agent such as chloramine T. Addition of glucose oxidase (EC 1.1.3.4) which generates hydrogen peroxide from glucose in situ, still further minimises the potential for damage (Miyachi et al., 1972). Furthermore, a reducing agent is not required since simple dilution will stop the reaction. Alternatively, the lactoperoxidase can be attached to a solid-phase and removed by centrifugation (Karonen et al., 1975). It has been claimed that tracers prepared by this technique suffer less 'damage' than those prepared by the chloramine T method (Thorell and Johansson, 1971; Karonen et al., 1975) and that no free iodine is released into the solution. The procedure is therefore often used where tracer with minimal alteration is essential (e.g., in radioreceptor assays). However, rigorous comparison with fully optimised methods using small amounts of chloramine T have shown little or no difference between the two methods when applied to small peptides (Heber et al., 1978) and a similar comparison for other materials has yet to be published. The disadvantage of lactoperoxidase is that the preparation of the reagents and the conditions for the reaction itself are more technically demanding than those for the chloramine T procedure. A typical procedure for lactoperoxidase iodination is shown in Table 3.3 (Nielsen et al., 1979).

3.7.1.3. 'Iodogen' (Fraker and Speck, 1978) A sparingly soluble oxidising agent (1,3,4,6-tetrachloro-3α,6α-diphenyl-glycouril) is evaporated on to the walls of a reaction vessel from a solution in methylene chloride. The material to be iodinated and ^{125}I are added. The reaction is terminated when the mixture is removed from the vessel without requiring addition of reducing agent.

3.7.1.4. Conjugation labelling In this procedure a carrier molecule is used: the carrier includes a phenol or imidazole group capable of iodination, and an amine group which can be directly coupled to carboxyl groups on the ligand or its derivatives (Bolton and Hunter, 1972, 1973) (Fig. 3.4, 3.5 and Table 3.4). Carriers are also available for conjugation to amine groups on the ligand (e.g., flurorescein isothiocyanate, N-acetyl-l-

TABLE 3.3

Iodination using solid-phase lactoperoxidase (Nielsen et al., 1979)

(general procedure for any protein)

Diluent buffer: Phosphate 0.1 M (pH 7.4) with *no* added protein*
1. Dissolve purified protein (5 μg) in 0.01 ml buffer in a small conical vial.
2. Add 0.3 ml buffer.
3. Add 1 mCi carrier-free sodium ^{125}I (volume approx. 0.01 ml).
4. Add 0.01 ml solid-phase lactoperoxidase** and 0.005 ml hydrogen peroxide solution.***
5. After 10 min add a further 0.005 ml hydrogen peroxide.****
6. After a further 20 min (total iodination time 30 min) add 0.1 ml buffer containing 0.1 g% sodium azide and then 0.1 ml buffer containing 1% bovine serum albumin.
7. Centrifuge at 1000 g at room temperature for 1 min.
8. Aspirate the supernatant and transfer to a column for purification (see Table 3.5 for example).

---

* None of the reagents should contain enzyme inhibitors such as sodium azide or reducing agents
** The solid-phase lactoperoxidase is prepared by linking 5 mg lactoperoxidase (Grade B, Calbiochem) to 10 mg maleic anhydride butanediol divinylether copolymer (Merck or British Drug Houses) according to the method of Karonen and his colleagues (1975). The final preparation is stored in 7 ml of 0.01 M acetate buffer (pH 5) and is stable for 1–2 years at 4°C. The optimal amount of lactoperoxidase may differ between preparations, and can be established by pilot experiments using different amounts of the solid-phase enzyme. The aim should be a 90–95% incorporation of iodide into tracer
*** Prepared by diluting 0.01 ml hydrogen peroxide (100 vol.) to 100 ml with distilled water, then a further 10-fold dilution (0.1–1 ml with distilled water). Note that the concentration of hydrogen peroxide is critical and ideally should be equimolar to the ^{125}I. Excess amounts can inhibit the enzyme
**** This second addition of H_2O_2 is necessary only if experience shows that yields are sub-optimal (i.e., < 90%)

histidine; Gavel and Shapiro, 1978; Kamel et al., 1979). The carrier may be iodinated either before or after conjugation to the ligand.

The conjugation technique has several advantages:

(1) It does not expose the ligand to the chemical damage associated with conventional iodination reactions;

(2) It can be applied to peptides which do not have tyrosine residues;

(3) The final reaction, mixing of the peptide and the iodinated ester, is very simple.

(4) The largest application is to non-peptide materials (e.g., the steroid hormones) which cannot be iodinated directly.

The disadvantages are:

(1) The substituted label, being considerably larger than the iodine atom, may lead to physicochemical alteration of the tracer;

(2) With haptens such as steroids and drugs, the label may bind well to antibody but fail to be displaced by unlabelled material, i.e. a 'flat' standard curve; this is because the antiserum contains populations of high-affinity antibodies directed towards the bridge between the hapten and the tag (Fig. 3.6); in some cases this problem can be overcome by appropriate selection of an antiserum (see Jeffcoate,

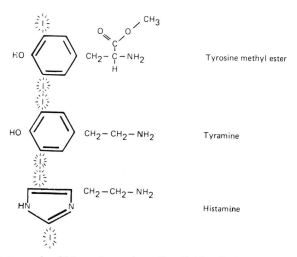

Fig. 3.4. Compounds which can be used as a 'handle' for the indirect attachment of ^{125}I to the ligand.

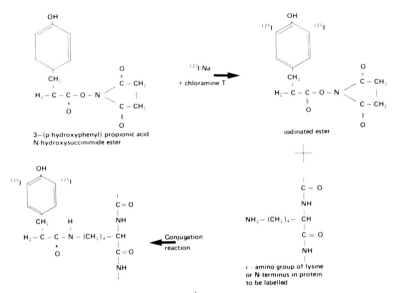

Fig. 3.5. Scheme of the conjugation labelling technique of Bolton and Hunter (1973).

1978), or by using disequilibrium conditions (Niswender, 1980), or by choosing different bridges for the immunogen and the tracer (England et al., 1974; Nordblom et al., 1981);

(3) Iodotyrosine or iodohistamine may itself bind to serum proteins, especially thyroxine-binding globulin, and thus lead to artefacts in unextracted samples (Painter and Vader, 1979).

3.7.2. Choice of iodination procedure

Some protein molecules are simple to iodinate and the products are robust. For these all methods are equally suitable; growth hormone is a good example (Apinyacharti and Baxter, 1979). Other molecules are difficult to iodinate and the products are unstable; ferritin is particularly notorious in this respect. Between these extremes all possible variations may be found and the best method has to be found by experience,

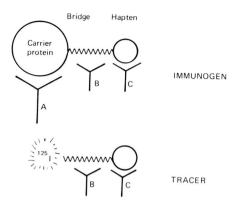

Fig. 3.6. A problem with the conjugation labelling of small molecules (haptens). The antiserum will contain populations of antibodies directed to the carrier protein (A), the hapten (C) and the bridge between the two (B). If the tracer contains the same bridge then it will be firmly bound by antibodies to the bridge, and cannot be displaced by pure hapten (i.e., standard or endogenous material). Greatest sensitivity is achieved when the bridge is dissimilar to that in the immunogen, but unfortunately specificity is often best when the label and immunogen are similar (Rowell et al., 1979).

bearing in mind that different preparations of the same molecule may vary in their iodination properties.

As a rule of thumb, chloramine T should be tried first. If this is not satisfactory, then attempts should be made with iodogen or lactoperoxidase. Finally, with the most refractory protein molecules, conjugation labelling may be the only suitable method. Iodination of haptens such as steroids represent a special case where various forms of conjugation labelling are the only possible approach.

3.7.3. Practical aspects of chloramine T iodination

A protocol for the iodination of a 'typical' peptide by the chloramine T technique is shown in Table 3.5. The exact conditions for a given substance may vary from those shown, but certain general principles can be stated:

TABLE 3.4

General method for conjugation labelling of proteins

(from Bolton and Hunter, 1973)*

---

1. Open a vial containing 1 mCi iodinated ester shown in Fig. 3.5 [*N*-succinidimyl 3-(4-hydroxy,5-[^{125}I]iodophenyl) propionate] (Radiochemical Centre, Code No. IM 861)** and evaporate solvent by directing a gentle stream of nitrogen on to the surface.
2. Add protein (5 μg) in 0.01 ml 0.1 M borate buffer (pH 8.5) and agitate for 15 min at 0°C.
3. Add 0.5 ml of 0.2 M glycine in 0.1 M borate buffer (pH 8.5) for 5 min at 0°C (the glycine reacts with the unchanged ester and prevents subsequent conjugation to carrier proteins).
4. Purify the reaction mixture on a column of Sephadex G-50 or G-75, and assess tracer (see Tables 3.5, 3.6 and Fig. 3.10, 3.11, 3.12).

---

* The method was originally described for hGH but is likely to be suitable for all proteins. Though the iodophenols are the most widely used, the iodohistamines have been advocated by some because of their greater stability (Tantchou and Slaunwhite, 1979)
** Considerable product variation has been noted between different manufacturers. Unfortunately, the suitability for a given application can only be established by trial and error

(1) *Choice of isotope*: ^{125}I is preferred to ^{131}I because:

(*i*) The half-life is greater (60 days against 8 days);

(*ii*) The counting efficiency in a 2 in. well-type crystal is greater;

(*iii*) The isotopic abundance (number of radioactive atoms relative to non-radioactive atoms (^{127}I)) is greater for current preparations of ^{125}I (100% against 20%);

(*iv*) The radiation emitted by ^{125}I is less penetrating than that of ^{131}I and thus presents less radiation hazard.

Because of the obvious superiority of ^{125}I, the only present use for ^{131}I is in assays using two tracers for the simultaneous measurement of two separate molecules (e.g., LH and FSH).

(2) *Concentration of reagents*:   The concentration of all reagents in the reaction mixture should be as high as possible. Since the absolute amounts are determined by other factors, this means using the smallest possible

TABLE 3.5

Preparation of an iodinated protein by chloramine T for radioimmunoassay

(iodinated hPL)

Diluent buffer: Phosphate 0.05 M (pH 7.4) with *no* added protein.

1. Dissolve purified hPL (50 μg) in 0.02 ml buffer in a small conical vial. It is convenient to prepare aliquots of this type for iodination by freeze-drying the appropriate volume of a solution of hPL in a series of such vials.
2. Add 2 mCi carrier-free Na^{125}I (volume about 0.02 ml) (obtained from the Radiochemical Centre, Amersham, code IMS30, or similar supplier).
3. Add chloramine T (10 μg) in 0.02 ml buffer. The solution should be freshly prepared immediately before the iodination.
4. Mix thoroughly but briefly (10–15 sec) by flicking with a finger; avoid splashing.
5. Immediately add sodium metabisulphite (20 μg) in 0.02 ml buffer. Mix.
6. Add 0.5 ml diluent buffer containing 2 mg/ml bovine serum albumin.
7. Transfer carefully to a 1 x 15 cm (about) column of Sephadex G-75, previously washed with diluent buffer containing 2 mg/ml bovine serum albumin.
8. Elute with same diluent buffer. Collect fractions of about 0.5 ml.
9. Assess tracer as shown in Table 3.6.
10. Store tracer as deep-frozen aliquots.

Comments: The procedure outlined has a wide range of possible variations, particularly in the relative amounts of label and protein. However, certain general points should be stated:

(*i*) The volumes of addition should be as small as possible in order to maintain high concentrations
(*ii*) The amount of chloramine T should be kept to a minimum
(*iii*) For this type of iodination, which yields one main protein peak and an iodide peak on gel filtration, the column can be relatively small. Total running time is around 30 min and the fractions can be collected manually. In cases where the protein fraction is very heterogeneous a larger column and running time is necessary

volumes; the total volume of the initial reaction mixture (isotope, peptide, chloramine T) should not usually exceed 100 μl.

(3) *Amount of chloramine T*: Since this is potentially damaging, the smallest possible amount should be used. Although traditionally 50 μg is used, it is often found that amounts of 10 μg or even 2 μg are equally effective and that the resulting product shows less damage and is more stable on storage. The minimum required can only be established by trial and error.

(4) *pH of reagents*:   The optimal pH for iodination of tyrosine residues is 7.5; above pH 8 there is a tendency for other groups to be substituted and above pH 9 the reaction becomes highly inefficient. Since iodine isotopes are usually supplied as a solution in 0.1 N NaOH, the composition of the other reactants must be such as to buffer this to pH 7.5.

(5) *Mixing of reagents*:   One of the commonest faults leading to poor yields is inadequate mixing of reagents. This is especially the case when small volumes are used: a small drop on the wall of the tube, which is not shaken down into the reaction mixture, may represent 50% or more of one of the reactants.

(6) *Speed of mixing*:   For the concentrations shown in Table 3.5, the iodination reaction is virtually instantaneous. Mixing should, therefore, only continue for long enough to ensure that mixing has indeed occurred. The whole process, from addition of primary reagents until the reaction is stopped by the addition of reducing agent, should not occupy more than 20-30 sec.

(7) *Temperature of reaction*:   Some workers prefer to carry out iodination with reagents cooled in ice. No consistent advantage over operation at room temperature has been demonstrated.

(8) *Quality of the isotope*:   It is traditional when an iodination has failed to attribute this to poor 'quality' of the isotope. When the iodine isotopes first became widely available there was considerable variation from batch to batch, but in recent years the situation has improved to the point where failure of an iodination is virtually never due to the isotope itself; almost invariably, the problem can be traced to one or more simple mistakes in the technical procedure.

3.7.4. Iodination damage

'Damage' can be simply defined as that fraction of the tracer ligand which will not react with the binder. This is a practical and operational defintion, which does not take into account any of a variety of physico-chemical alterations which are not reflected by the performance of the tracer in the assay. There are several possible causes of damage as defined above.

(1) *Alteration of the molecule by the presence of an iodine atom*:   In principle, the addition of iodine may affect the reactivity of a smaller molecule more than that of a larger molecule. Thus oestrogens, iodinated through their phenolic A ring, will no longer react with specific antisera. Under other circumstances, the label may alter only part of the molecule, affecting the specificity of the system. This is illustrated by the hypothetical situation shown in Fig. 3.7.

Three methods are available for the comparison of labelled and unlabelled ligand:

(*i*) Comparison of iodinated material with material carrying an internal label such as ^3H; the practicality of this depends on the availability of the internally-labelled tracer;

(*ii*) Comparison with unlabelled ligand (Hunter, 1971): tubes are prepared containing a fixed amount of antibody and tracer; to one set is added serial dilutions of unlabelled ligand; to the other is added *identical* serial concentrations of tracer. If the tracer is 'undamaged', the tubes will contain identical amounts of total ligand and should yield superimposable curves;

(*iii*) Comparison of physicochemical properties of tracer and unlabelled ligand: as noted above, this will not necessarily reflect their behaviour in combination with the binder.

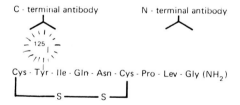

Fig. 3.7. How iodine substitution could affect the specificity of an assay, in this case that for the nonapeptide oxytocin. If the antiserum contains two populations of antibodies, directed to the C- and N-terminus of the molecule, respectively, and if the iodine completely alters the antigenicity of the N-terminus, then only the C-terminal antibodies will be effective in the assay. The assay would measure the intact molecule and C-terminal fragments of the molecule, but not N-terminal fragments.

(2) *Chemical damage*:   The peptide may be directly damaged by chemicals in the reaction mixture, most notably by oxidation or reduction. For example, even a mild oxidation procedure can partly split FSH into its α and β subunits, and thus affect the specificity of an assay (Marana et al., 1979). Other possible sources of chemical damage are less well-defined: for instance, that due to unidentified impurities in the isotope, or to an inherent instability of the peptide molecule in dilute solution in the absence of a carrier protein.

(3) *Internal radiation*:   The disintegration of an iodine atom may disrupt the molecule to which it is attached. Furthermore, the radiation emitted may lead to free radical formation during its passage through the aqueous solution and thus damage other molecules. Internal radiation is not thought to be a significant cause of damage in the relatively dilute solutions in which tracers are usually stored or used and can be virtually eliminated by incorporation of a free radical scavenger such as ethanol. It may, however, be important during the actual process of iodination when all reagents are at high concentration.

(4) *'Decay catastrophe' (Yalow and Berson, 1968)*:   This term describes the situation in which the decay of an attached iodine atom disrupts a molecule bearing another and as yet undecayed iodine atom (Fig. 3.8). The latter will then be attached to a molecular fragment which may no longer react with the binder but because it is still labelled will appear as 'damaged' tracer in the assay. This type of damage can only occur with

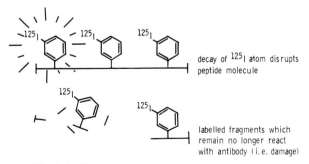

Fig. 3.8. The mechanism of 'decay catastrophe'.

molecules containing at least two isotopic iodine atoms and is therefore a characteristic of high specific activity tracers. Both decay catastrophe and internal radiation are responsible for the familiar observation that such tracers have the shortest shelf-life in terms of damage. Since in most assays, adequate specific activity can be achieved by a substitution level of one atom of iodine per molecule or less, higher levels should be avoided whenever possible.

(5) *Incubation damage*:   Tracer ligand may be progressively destroyed during the assay procedure itself because of the presence of damaging agents in the incubation mixture. This can lead to artefactual results. If, for example, 50% of the tracer is rendered non-reactive, the final result will be identical to that obtained in the presence of a concentration of unlabelled ligand sufficient to produce a 50% reduction in total binding. To the unwary this might be interpreted as an actual level of the un-labelled ligand. Examples of this situation and means for its avoidance are given in § 10.3.3.

(6) *Impurity damage*:   So-called 'pure' antigen used for iodination may be contaminated with irrelevant material which, since it takes up label but does not react with the binder must be described as 'damage'. The presence of such contaminants may already be known from physico-chemical studies on the 'pure' antigen. However, these studies can be misleading when the methods available for the detection of the contaminants (e.g., spectrophotometry) are considerably less sensitive than their detection as radioactive tracers. This situation is shown diagrammatically in Fig. 3.9.

(7) *Iodine release*:   With many labelled materials there appears to be a progressive release of free iodide on storage. The rate of 'deiodination' varies with different iodination procedures, and is probably greatest in preparations containing substituents other than monoiodotyrosine (Krohn, et al., 1977).

3.7.5. *Purification of iodinated tracer*

When the iodination is complete the reaction mixture contains the following: unlabelled ligand (damaged and undamaged); labelled ligand

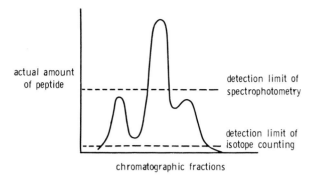

chromatographic fractions

Fig. 3.9. How a protein can seem to consist of a single component when examined by an insensitive technique (spectrophotometry), and of multiple components when examined after iodination by a sensitive technique (isotope counting). The extra peaks might be attributed to 'damage' when in fact they were present in the original preparation.

(damaged and undamaged); free iodide; and salts including the oxidising and reducing agent. Since the tracer used in the assay should consist of not less than 95% undamaged labelled ligand, and since the proportion in the reaction mixture is usually much less, a purification procedure is essential.

Virtually all of the physicochemical separation procedures which are used in protein and peptide chemistry have been applied to the purification of iodinated tracer. The criteria for a purification procedure are that it should be efficient, simple and rapid. Each of the possible procedures will be briefly noted, though the only technique commonly used is gel-filtration chromatography.

(1) *Dilution*:   It is customary to dilute the iodination mixture as soon as the primary reactions are complete. Although dilution cannot be truly described as purification, it does serve specific purposes:
   (*i*) It provides sufficient volume to make subsequent handling relatively easy.
   (*ii*) It reduces the possibility of damage due to internal radiation or the presence of high concentrations of chemical agents.

(*iii*) It is usual to include a protein such as albumin in the diluent which serves as a carrier and obviates the instability of many proteins in very dilute solution.

(2) *Chemical precipitation*:   This might, for example, be applied to the separation of iodinated IgG from free iodide, by precipitation of the former with half a volume of saturated ammonium sulphate. In practice it is little if ever used because it can easily lead to damaged products.

(3) *Dialysis*:   Although this would separate most peptides from iodide, it has several disadvantages including the relatively long time which is necessary, the absorption of many peptides to dialysis membranes, and the fact that it will not readily separate damaged from undamaged material.

(4) *Adsorption*:   In its simplest form this consists of the batchwise addition of an ion-exchange resin to the diluted reaction mixture, thus removing free iodide and salts. This is of value only with those materials where damaged labelled peptide is relatively insignificant. For larger peptides, such as ACTH and gonadotrophins, use has been made of particulate adsorbents such as cellulose, employed either batchwise or in the form of a small column. However, the process is ill-understood and success may vary with different batches of adsorbent.

(5) *Ion-exchange chromatography*:   This is a sophisticated procedure which with the use of appropriate gradients can readily separate minor variants of a peptide, including damaged and undamaged matter, uniodinated and iodinated material (Heber et al., 1978). It is relatively little used in practice because it can be time-consuming and laborious.

(6) *Group-specific adsorbent chromatography*:   Concanavalin A linked to agarose (Con A-Sepharose, Pharmacia) selectively binds molecules containing carbohydrates, including glycoproteins. Absorption to a matrix of this type, followed by elution with α-methyl-D-glucoside, may considerably improve the immunoreactivity of materials such as iodinated TSH (Nisula et al., 1978).

(7) *Gel-filtration chromatography*: This is the most widely applied technique for the purification of iodinated tracers. The detailed procedure does not differ greatly from other applications (see Fischer, 1980), though speed becomes an important criterion because the aim should be to prepare and characterise a tracer within a 24 h period. The choice of column size and material will vary with the ligand. If the intention is to separate reasonably homogeneous, labelled material from free iodide then a relatively small column (e.g., 10 cm x 0.5 cm) of a low porosity gel (Sephadex G-25 or G-50) is adquate. However, if the tracer is likely to be heterogeneous then a rather larger column is necessary (e.g.,

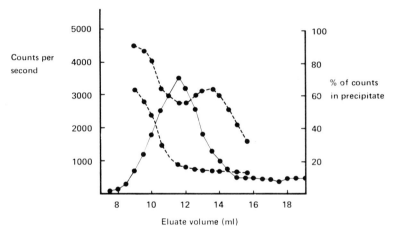

Fig. 3.10. Chromatography of iodinated pregnancy-specific β_1-glycoprotein (M_r 80 000) on a 40 cm x 1 cm column of Sephadex G-200 eluted with phosphate buffer containing 1 mg/ml of bovine serum albumin. There is a single but rather broad peak of radioactive protein (•——•) (the free iodide peak appeared in later fractions and is not shown here). A small aliquot from each fraction was incubated with and without an excess of antibody, and the bound fraction was precipitated with 20% polyethylene glycol (see Table 6.3). The interrupted lines (•– – –•) show the per cent of counts precipitated in the presence (upper line) and absence (lower line) of antibody. The earliest fractions give very high blank values, probably due to the presence of aggregates, and would not be suitable for use in an assay. The best fractions are those on the trailing edge of the protein peak which give the highest antibody bound levels in the presence of a relatively low blank. (Data kindly supplied by A.T.M. Al-Ani.)

40 cm x 1 cm; see Fig. 3.10) and a gel of high porosity (Sephadex G-75, G-100 or G-200). As a general rule, larger columns are always desirable with iodinated proteins because these will almost inevitably show some degree of heterogeneity (Fig. 3.10 and 3.11). Further improvements may be possible with the newer 'high-resolution' gels (e.g., the Ultrogel series (Pharmacia)).

The assessment of a tracer after purification by gel filtration is summarised in Table 3.6.

(8) *Thin-layer chromatography*:   This is widely used in the purification of tracer ligands of low M_r, such as steroids and certain drugs (Stahl, 1969).

(9) *Electrophoresis*:   This is little used because simple two-dimensional systems (paper or cellulose acetate) can only accept very limited quantities of material; three-dimensional systems (starch-gel or polyacrylamide-gel) will accept larger loads, but are laborious to perform. With starch-

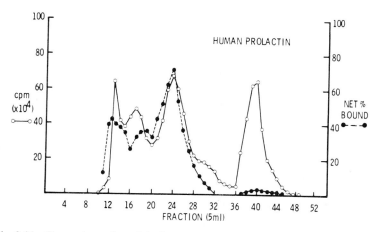

Fig. 3.11. Chromatography of iodinated human prolactin on a 10 cm x 1 cm column of Sephadex G-75 eluted with 60 mM barbitone buffer containing 0.5 mg/ml human serum albumin. The first three peaks represent protein, and the fourth peak free iodide. Of the three protein peaks only the third showed any significant reaction with a specific antibody to prolactin.

gel electrophoresis, separation and purification of ^{131}I-labelled insulin on the basis of the level of iodine substitution has been demonstrated (Berson and Yalow, 1966) and similar separations have been achieved with isoelectric focussing (Dermody et al., 1979). Although of considerable value in the initial development of an assay, these procedures are little used in practice.

(10) *Immunopurification*:   A tracer could be purified from the initial reaction mixture by exposure to solid-phase antibody (see § 6.3.6.2), followed by appropriate washes and elution. This approach has been little used because it would demand relatively large amounts of solid-phase antibody. However, a comparable approach is used in the immunoradiometric assay (Miles and Hales, 1968) in which purified antibody is iodinated while actually in combination with solid-phase antigen (see § 6.4).

The preparation and purification of an iodinated tracer should not, if possible, occupy more than a working day, since tracer allowed to remain at room temperature will deteriorate more rapidly than that which is deep frozen. The conditions for the storage of a tracer are similar to those for storage of solutions of standard (see § 2.6). In particular, it should be stored in aliquots such that it is never necessary to freeze and thaw the solution more than once. In any one laboratory, iodinated material should be kept in a freezer designated specifically for that purpose; the freezer should be placed as far as possible from working areas and counters.

Because of the possibility of progressive damage to the labelled antigen some workers repurify each stored aliquot by chromatography after it is thawed for use. This is undoubtedly effective, but very time-consuming for a routine assay.

3.7.6. Chemical assessment of tracer

A freshly prepared tracer must be carefully assessed both chemically, and by its behaviour in the assay (see Table 3.6). Chemical assessment is designed to ascertain three characteristics of the iodination: the yield, the specific activity of the tracer, and the absolute concentration of the tracer. 'Yield' is defined as the percentage incorporation of the isotope into labelled peptide; this calculation does not usually take into account damaged or undamaged forms of the peptide. 'Specific activity of the tracer' is defined as the radioactivity per unit mass or mole of ligand (e.g., mCi/μg); for practical reasons this calculation again does not usually distinguish between damaged and undamaged. 'Concentration of the tracer' is simply mass per unit volume. Despite the importance of this parameter to assay design, its calculation is all too frequently ignored and the tracer distributed as 'counts' rather than concentration. In those situations in which the proportion of damaged tracer is high, appropriate corrections should be applied in calculating concentration so that the value refers only to undamaged materials.

All three parameters can be calculated from the results of the physico-chemical purification procedure (Fig. 3.12). Additional analytical procedures are sometimes used and include:

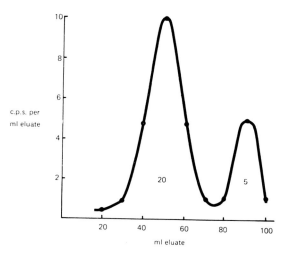

Fig. 3.12. Theoretical example to illustrate calculation of yield, specific activity, and tracer concentration after chromatography of an iodinated protein. There are 20 'counts' in the protein peak (first) and 5 in the later iodide peak. Thus the yield is 20/25 or 80%. Assuming that the amount of protein iodinated was 10 μg and the amount of ^{125}I used was 1 mCi the specific activity is 80 μCi/μg. The protein peak has a volume of 40 ml and the concentration of the pooled tracer is 0.25 μg/ml.

(1) *Electrophoresis*: The most familiar technique is 'chromatoelectrophoresis' (Berson et al., 1956) which separates both free iodide and damaged from undamaged components;

(2) *'Wick chromatography' (Orskov, 1967)*: An aliquot of the iodination mixture is spotted on to a narrow strip of paper one end of which is placed in a 10% solution of trichloracetic acid. As this solution migrates up the strip the iodinated protein is precipitated and remains at its origin. Free iodide and small damaged products such as iodotyrosine and iodopeptides are not precipitated and thus move with the solvent front, giving a clear separation from the tracer.

Although the calculation of yield, specific activity, and concentration of tracer is relatively simple, certain provisos should be noted. Considerable losses may occur at different steps of the procedure: for example, by absorption on to surfaces such as those of the pipettes, the reaction vessel, and the matrix of any material used for purification. These losses may approach 50%. To some extent they can be corrected by counting the residual radioactivity of the containers after use. However, with the exception of the pipette used for delivery of isotope, the nature of the retained radioactivity cannot easily be specified, and might represent proportions of free iodide and labelled peptide which differ widely from those present in the final preparation. This may explain why calculation of the yield from the results of two different separation procedures can give discrepant answers. A further problem may arise with procedures which separate damaged and undamaged tracer: calculation of specific activity and concentration of the undamaged form is based on the assumption that the level of iodine substitution is equivalent for both forms. This assumption may be false: a small peak of radioactivity might represent a very large amount of protein with relatively few iodine atoms per molecule.

The final calculation which can be of great value in the initial setting-up of an assay is to estimate the number of iodine atoms per molecule of ligand. This can be worked out from the specific activity expressed in molar terms, where the specific activity of ^{125}I at 100% isotopic abundance is approximately 1.8 mCi/nmol. For example, assume that 20 μg of a peptide hormone of M_r 20 000, such as hPL, hCG or prolactin, is iodinated with 2 mCi of ^{125}I, giving a yield of 90%. Ninety per cent of 2 mCi is 1.8 mCi, equivalent to 1 nmol of iodine; 20 mg of the hormone is also equivalent to 1 nmol. The level of substitution is therefore one atom of iodine per molecule of hormone. A calculation of this type can be of great practical value. All other things being equal, substitution of one atom per molecule can be regarded as the optimum; higher levels may alter the immunoreactivity of a molecule, and are indicative of disubstitution and consequent decay catastrophe (see § 3.7.4); lower levels are unnecessary since the tracer will simply be diluted by unlabelled ligand molecules.

3.7.7. Immunological assessment of tracer

This is much the most important aspect of the evaluation of a newly prepared tracer, and consists simply of testing an aliquot of the pooled

TABLE 3.6
Assessment of an iodinated protein for radioimmunoassay

1. Collect an aliquot (5–10 μl) from each fraction of the protein peak from the Sephadex column (Table 3.5) (see Fig. 3.10, 3.11, 3.12).
2. Dilute each aliquot in diluent buffer with 3 mg/ml bovine serum albumin such that 0.2 ml yields about 10 000 counts in 10 sec.
3. Incubate each aliquot with and without an excess of antiserum, using conditions identical with those of the '0' standard and assay blank (Table 1.3 and Fig. 1.7).
4. Combine those fractions containing the most immunoreactive materials, and store.
5. If experience over a series of iodinations shows that certain fractions invariably give the best performance, then in a routine iodination, these fractions can be pooled prior to testing.

The following data should be recorded (see Fig. 3.10, 3.11, 3.12):
1. A graph of the counts eluted from the column.
2. Plotted on the same graph, the percentage of each fraction bound in antibody excess.
3. The yield (%) calculated from the elution pattern ([total counts in protein peak/total counts eluted] × 100).
4. The concentration of tracer ligand in the combined fractions (total amount of ligand used/volume of protein fractions; if a substantial amount of the protein peak is rejected allowance must be made for this).

Additional methods of assessment are discussed in the main text (§ 3.7.6 and 3.7.7). These have, as their object, the detailed assessment of a tracer during the development stage of an assay.

tracer for binding in the presence and absence of antibody (see Table 3.6). The results are compared with those of previous iodinations to determine whether the performance is acceptable in terms of assay blank and maximum binding. On rare occasions these parameters may not be an adequate guide to performance in the assay, in which case a standard curve and quality controls will have to be included as part of the assessment procedure. At this stage of development of an assay it is useful to test each individual fraction following chromatography: very often this will reveal heterogeneity within the protein peak itself, and thus suggest that only selected fractions should be pooled for use in the assay (see Fig. 3.10 and 3.11).

3.8. Variations on the use of radiolabelled tracers

3.8.1. Universal tracers

Staphylococcal protein A can bind specifically to the Fc region of immunoglobulin molecules and has been used in the separation of bound and free ligand (see § 6.3.3.3). An ingenious use of this material is as a 'universal tracer' (Langone, 1978): antibody and ligand are incubated in liquid phase; solid-phase ligand is then added and absorbs 'free' antibody; finally the amount of antibody on the solid phase is quantitated by addition of ^{125}I-labelled protein A.

Another ingenious suggestion for a universal tracer is the use of immunopurified ^{125}I-labelled antibodies to 2,4-dinitrophenyl (DNP). The primary antibody is labelled with DNP, and the anti-DNP is then used as a tracer for bound antibody in a two-site immunometric system (see § 6.4).

3.8.2. Autoradiographic radioimmunoassay

A system has been described in which the assay is performed in a multi-well test-plate. After separation of bound and free ligand the plate is exposed to X-ray film; the size and density of the resulting spots reflects the amount of radioactivity (Weiler and Zenk, 1979). This procedure is less precise than conventional techniques but has good potential for assays in which a semi-quantitative result is required.

3.8.3. Internal sample attenuators

A radioimmunoassay for T3 has been described in which the free fraction is absorbed to charcoal co-immobilised in starch spheres with bismuth oxide (Eriksson, Mattiasson and Thorell, 1981). The latter effectively 'shields' the radioactive emission of the free phase and thus permits counting of the bound phase without separation – a principle similar to that of the homogeneous non-isotopic assays (see Ch. 4).

3.8.4. Liposome immune assay

Antigens are inserted into iodine or fluorescein-labelled lipid vesicles which can then be precipitated by antiserum; this has been applied to transplantation antigens (Axelsson et al., 1981).

CHAPTER 4

Requirements for binding assays – tracer ligand using non-isotopic labels

Any material which can be accurately determined at low levels, and which can be firmly attached to the ligand molecule without grossly altering its properties, may serve as a label. Examples are shown in Table 4.1. The principle advantages of non-isotopic over isotopic labels are:
(1) They have a prolonged shelf-life, and thus avoid many problems of distribution and storage;
(2) They do not constitute a radiation hazard;
(3) Because the properties of the label may differ strikingly in the bound and free phases a separation step is often not necessary and the procedures should be readily adaptable to automation (see Ch. 13).
The principle disadvantages of non-isotopic labels are:
(1) End-point detection may be less precise than that of nuclear counting (this is certainly the case for enzymes, but probably not for fluorescent labels); and
(2) Materials with properties similar to the label may occur as normal components of a biological sample and thus yield background 'noise' which severely limits both sensitivity and precision. This is probably the major stumbling block to the rapid replacement of all isotopic procedures with the superficially very attractive non-isotopic alternatives.

TABLE 4.1
Materials which can serve as label for the tracer in a binding assay

Isotopes	Chemiluminescent molecules
Particles	Bioluminescent systems
Enzymes (and cofactors)	Bacteriophages
Fluorogenic molecules	Metals (Cais et al., 1977; Leuvering et al., 1980)
Free radicals (Leute et al., 1972)	

It cannot be emphasized too strongly that the introduction of a non-isotopic label is not a panacea which eliminates the need for careful attention to all other aspects of reagent choice and assay design. With the exception, in some cases, of the need for a separation step, the criteria for any system remain exactly those for any binding assay as set out in other chapters.

4.1. Particle labels

It is not often appreciated that many of the classical agglutination methods in immunology are, in fact, variants of binding assays in which the label is a particle. The most commonly used pregnancy tests, in which latex particles coated with antiserum to hCG agglutinate in the presence of hCG, are a good example of this. Indeed, the haemagglutination-inhibition assay for insulin described by Arquilla and Stavitsky in 1956 differed from the later developed radioimmunoassays only in the choice of a red cell rather than an isotope as the label.

Particle label techniques are usually qualitative rather than quantitative, i.e. they give a yes or no answer depending on whether or not agglutination has occurred. Intermediate stages may be read by eye but the results are very subjective. Recently, however, instrumentation has become available for particle sizing and counting which holds the promise of quantitation comparable to that achieved with other labels. For example, a thyroxine (T_4) assay has been described in which the antigen is linked to dextran and the antibody is coated on to latex particles (Cambiaso et al., 1977) (Technicon 'PACIA' system); in the absence of unlabelled T_4 the latter will agglutinate with the T_4–dextran conjugate. In the presence of T_4 this process is blocked, and the number of free particles increases in direct proportion to the amount of T_4 present. Though excellent sensitivity can be achieved by procedures of this type, they are very susceptible to non-specific interference by factors present in biological samples such as serum.

4.2. Enzyme labels (enzymoimmunoassay, EIA)

These are currently the most widely used of non-isotopic labels. Because of the catalytic nature of enzyme activity, a single molecule of an enzyme may be responsible for the conversion of many molecules of substrate. Thus, small quantities of enzyme can be quantitated by studying substrate conversion using simple and relatively insensitive techniques such as colorimetry. Since specific enzymes can readily be coupled to other molecules by covalent links (Appendix VI), they can be used as labels for the production of tracer. This possibility has now been demonstrated for a variety of materials (Van Weemen and Schuurs, 1971; Wisdom, 1976; Scharpe et al., 1976; Landon et al., 1979; O'Sullivan et al., 1979) and using a wide range of enzyme labels (Table 4.2). Co-enzymes (e.g., nicotine or

TABLE 4.2
Enzymes in common use for enzymoimmunoassay

The criterion is that the enzymes must be stable and have high activity at a pH which does not disturb the antigen–antibody reaction. Enzymes for homogeneous systems must be very resistant to non-specific interference from serum

	Classification
Heterogeneous EIA	
Horseradish peroxidase	(EC 1.11.1.17)
Alkaline phosphatase	(EC 3.1.3.1)
β-D-Galactosidase	(EC 3.2.1.23)
Glucose oxidase	(EC 1.1.3.4)
Glucoamylase	(EC 3.2.1.3)
Carbonic anhydrase	(EC 4.2.1.1)
Acetylcholinesterase	(EC 3.1.1.7)
Catalase	(EC 1.11.1.6)
Penicillinase	(EC 3.5.2.6)
Homogeneous EIA	
Lysozyme	(EC 3.2.1.17)
Malate dehydrogenase	(EC 1.1.1.37)
Glucose 6-phosphate dehydrogenase	(EC 1.1.1.49)
β-D-Galactosidase	(EC 3.2.1.23)

TABLE 4.3
Types of enzymoimmunoassay (EIA)

Type of assay	Principle
Heterogeneous EIA	Enzyme replaces isotope label
Immunoenzymatic assay (IEMA)	Enzyme replaces isotopic label on antibody
Homogeneous EIA (Enzyme multiplied immunoassay technique, EMIT)	Enzyme activity quenched in bound fraction
Homogeneous EIA (enzyme enhancement)	Enzyme activity enhanced in bound fraction

flavine adenine dinucleotide) can also be used as label, the activity being reduced in the antibody-bound fraction (Kohen et al., 1979; Morris et al., 1981). The various types of enzymoimmunoassay are described in Table 4.3. Enzyme labels can be used in exactly the same manner as isotopic labels, with a procedure, in some systems, to separate bound and free phases following incubation. They also offer the opportunity, not available with isotopes, for elimination of the separation procedure. The former systems are often referred to as 'heterogeneous', and those not requiring separation as 'homogeneous'. Detection systems include simple colorimetry, measurement of heat production (Mattiasson et al., 1978), use of ion-specific electrodes directly interfaced to solid-phase antibody (Boitieux et al., 1979), chemiluminescence induced by peroxidase (Velan and Halman, 1978), spectrofluorimetry (Kate et al., 1979), and conversion of radioactive substrates (Harris et al., 1979).

4.2.1. Heterogeneous enzymoimmunoassays

These differ from RIA in the end-point detection system, and in the fact that the range of separation procedures is limited to second antibody or solid-phase because, unlike isotopes, there may be little difference between bound and free phases in terms of molecular weight and charge. The separation procedure serves an additional and important function with EIA since it separates the exogenous enzyme label from endogenous enzymes (or inhibitors) in the sample; the latter will otherwise give a high level of background 'noise' which severely limits the sensitivity of the assay. Reduction in noise with multiple wash steps in an EIA can yield assays with sensitivity in the pmol/l range, but the procedure is extremely cumbersome.

The first heterogeneous EIA were those for IgG (Engvall and Perlmann, 1971) and oestrogens (Van Weemen and Schuurs, 1971). Both used solid-phase antibody and were referred to as enzyme-linked immunosorbent assay (ELISA). Assays of this type have since been established for a wide range of haptens and proteins. Their specificity is similar to that of RIA, and they can achieve comparable sensitivity – for example, in the measurement of TSH at circulating levels in the range of pmol/l (Miyai et al., 1976; Kato et al., 1979). But they cannot achieve *greater* sensitivity, because this is limited almost entirely by the affinity of the antibody (see § 1.7). The reproducibility of EIA is almost certainly less than that of RIA because of the background noise due to endogenous enzymes in biological fluids (enzymes which are sufficiently robust to be used as a label are also those found in extracellular fluids); furthermore, enzyme determination is relatively imprecise when compared with isotope counting (Sun and Spihler, 1976; Galen and Forman, 1977; Weil et al., 1977). Thus the precision and sensitivity of EIA depends on the conditions of an enzyme–substrate interaction, the rate of which is a function of pH, substrate concentration, nature of substrate, enzyme activity of the conjugate, and temperature. Furthermore, the time dependence means that it is impossible to check a doubtful reading. With ELISA techniques, both reproducibility and practicality are also limited by the increased number of centrifugation and wash steps required. It seems likely that the best current applications of these procedures are for those substances which circulate at relatively high levels and in which the clinical problem requires a qualitative 'yes or no' rather than a quantitative answer (e.g., hepatitis B surface antigen, Wolters et al., 1976; Wei et al., 1977).

Enzymes can also be used to label the antibody in systems which are comparable to the immunoradiometric assay (IRMA) (see § 6.4) and which are referred to as 'immunoenzymatic assay' (IEMA) (Van Weemen and Schuurs, 1974; Maiolini et al., 1975). Assays of this type are now widely used for the detection of circulating antibodies to various infections. Two-site assays have also been described for larger molecules such as α-feto-protein (Belanger et al., 1973; Maiolini and Masseyeff, 1975). The advantages and problems of IEMA are similar to those of other heterogeneous enzymoimmunoassays.

4.2.2. Homogeneous enzymoimmunoassays

The best known of the homogeneous EIA's are those developed by the Syva Corporation and given the name 'enzyme multiplied immunoassay techniques' or 'EMIT'. In the most general procedure the enzyme is inactive of 'quenched' in the tracer–antibody complex, and activity can thus be measured in the free fraction without the need for a separation step (Rubenstein et al., 1972) (Fig. 4.1). The technique has been applied to a wide variety of drugs and has the advantage of speed, small sample volume (0.01 ml) or less, and good precision (between-assay variation of 10%). More recently, systems have been described in which enzyme activity is enhanced rather than quenched in the bound fraction (Ullman et al., 1975) (Fig. 4.2). This has been applied to the assay of thyroxine using a malate dehydrogenase label, and the assay lends itself well to automation (Galen and Forman, 1977).

Avoidance of the separation step greatly simplifies the assay by comparison with a heterogeneous system, and also partly compensates for the poor precision of end-point determination. However, sensitivity is much reduced by background noise due to endogenous enzyme activity in the sample; the limit is reached with compounds which circulate in the nmol/l range. Furthermore, homogeneous EIA cannot be applied to larger mole-

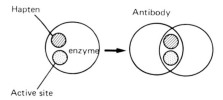

Fig. 4.1. The principle of 'quenching' enzymoimmunoassay. When the enzyme-labelled hapten is combined to the antibody the active site of the enzyme is masked by the antibody.

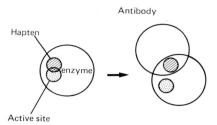

Fig. 4.2. The principle of 'enhancement' enzymoimmunoassay. In the free tracer the active site of the enzyme is masked by the hapten. In combination with antibody the active site is unmasked.

cules such as proteins, because the distance between the antigenic site and that of enzyme attachment is such that antibody binding will not usually affect enzyme activity.

4.3. Fluorescent labels (fluoroimmunoassay, FIA)

There are strong indications that the use of fluorescent compounds as labels may become one of the principle methods of 'non-isotopic' immunoassay. Thus, the lower limit of detection of a fluorescent tracer using standard equipment should permit the estimation of biological substances which circulate in the nanomolar range (e.g., thyroxine, cortisol, placental lactogen), while further developments will almost certainly extend this into the picomolar range. For this reason, fluorescent labels are considered in some detail here.

4.3.1. The nature and measurement of fluorescence

Fluorescence is the property of certain molecules ('fluorophores') to absorb light at one wavelength and emit a light at a longer wavelength. The incident light 'excites' the molecule to a higher level of vibrational energy: as the molecule returns to the ground state it emits a photon which is the fluorescence emission. Because of the rather complex nature of this reaction, both excitation and emission occur over a band of wavelengths referred to as the 'excitation spectrum' and the 'emission spectrum'. Both spectra have a maximum which is used to describe the properties of the molecule, and to define the optimum conditions for detection of the fluorescence. The gap between the excitation and emission maxima is referred to as the 'Stokes" shift (see Fig. 4.3); the relation between absorbed energy and emitted energy is known as the 'quantum efficiency' which has a theoretical maximum of 1.

The potential sensitivity of fluorescence determination is very high but in practice is often limited by background 'noise'. Noise can be due to either light scattering or the presence of fluorophores other than the label itself. Light scattering is essentially reflection of the incident light as it passes through the solution, either from solute molecules (Rayleigh scattering) or from particles in suspension (Tyndall scattering); obviously the wavelength of the scattered light is similar to that of the incident light and can be largely eliminated by appropriate choice of emission filters. A wide range of biological materials exhibit fluorescence and may be present in assay solution; these include both solute molecules and solvent molecules (the so-called Raman scattering). For example, whole serum fluoresces strongly with an excitation maximum of 340 nm and an emission maximum of 470 nm. Noise due to scattering or endogenous fluorophores can be reduced by attention to the characteristics of the fluorophore used as label. A large Stokes' shift (to eliminate scattering) and an emission maximum at a long wavelength (i.e., well beyond that of serum) are obviously desirable. In practice the choice will often be a compromise between specificity (noise reduction) and sensitivity (fluorescence inten-

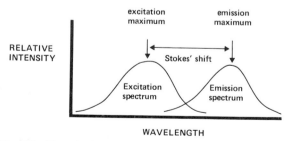

Fig. 4.3. The principle of fluorescence measurement (see text).

TABLE 4.4

Some fluorescent compounds (fluorophores) which may be of value in fluoro-immunoassay (for a detailed account see Soini and Hemmila, 1979)

Compound	Advantages	Disadvantages
Fluorescein	Widely used; high quantum efficiency	Relatively small Stokes' shift
Rhodamine	Fluorescence maximum at very long wavelengths	Quantum efficiency less than fluorescein
Dansyl	–	Low quantum efficiency; excitation and emission wavelengths similar to serum
Umbelliferyl	Large Stokes' shift	Quantum efficiency less than fluorescein
Rare-earth chelates	Large Stokes' shift; long decay times suitable for time-resolved fluorimeter	Low quantum efficiency

Note: Each compound is available as a number of derivatives (e.g., fluorescein isothiocyanate (FITC); dichlorotriazinyl fluorescein). The choice of derivative may influence the ease of coupling and stability and performance of the tracer

sity). The characteristics of some available fluorophores are shown in Table 4.4, but it should be noted that fluorescein isothiocyanate (FITC) is most commonly used.

Fluorescence is measured in a spectrofluorimeter which consists of a source of light, a sample holder, and a detector (Fig. 4.4). In current equipment the light source is usually a xenon-arc lamp, though other sources are possible; the detector is a simple photomultiplier tube. The wavelength of the excitation light and the emitted light is selected by the use of optical filters or diffraction grating monochromators. Filters are considerably cheaper and likely to be the method of choice for FIA. It is not appropriate here to consider fluorimeter design in greater detail, though this will be an important feature of the future development of FIA. Possible advances include:

(1) The introduction of simple, inexpensive equipment geared exclusively for use in FIA;

(2) The development of fast-throughput multi-detector systems similar to advanced γ-counters (see § 3.3);

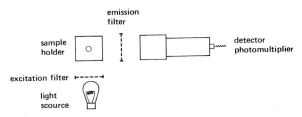

Fig. 4.4. The principal components of a spectrofluorimeter. The beam from the light source is resolved to a set wavelength by the excitation filter before it passes through the sample. Fluorescent light is emitted in all directions, and part falls on the emission filter/detector assembly which is set at a right-angle to the main beam.

(3) The use of lasers to provide a high intensity excitation beam (Gianturco et al., 1979; Lidofsky et al., 1979);

(4) The use of 'time-resolved' fluorimetry which separates fluorophores according to the decay-time of the excited stage – and thus permits precise and very specific quantitation of fluorophores with exceptionally long decay times, such as the chelates of rare earth metals (Soini and Hemmila, 1979);

(5) The use of polarisation fluorimetry – when a fluorescent molecule is excited with polarised light, the polarisation of the emitted light depends on the extent of random Brownian rotation of the molecules. With a small labelled antigen rotation is fast and the signal is small; after binding by antibody the signal is much enhanced (Dandliker et al., 1973);

(6) The use of photon counting to improve the signal-to-noise ratio of the detector system (Curry et al., 1979).

4.3.2. Types of fluoroimmunoassay (FIA)

As with EIA fluoroimmunoassay can be divided according to whether or not a separation step is required, i.e. heterogeneous or homogenous (Table 4.6). Heterogeneous FIA are comparable to RIA. Most of the common separation procedures can be used because of the relatively small M_r of fluorescein, but as with EIA, solid-phase systems are desirable because they permit removal of endogenous fluorophores. Heterogeneous FIA has

TABLE 4.5

Preparation of a fluoresceinated protein for use in fluoroimmunoassay (FIA) of hPL
(Chard and Sykes, 1979)

Diluent buffer: $Na_2HPO_4 \cdot 2 H_2O$, 0.15 M, (pH 9.5) with *no* added protein

1. Dissolve purified hPL (1 mg) in 0.25 ml buffer.
2. Add 0.1 ml of a solution (1 mg/ml) of fluorescein isothiocyanate (FITC; Calbiochem) in the same buffer.
3. If necessary, adjust pH to 9.5 by addition of 1 M Tris.
4. Mix and stand for 2 h at room temperature.
5. Transfer carefully to a 8 × 90 mm (approx.) column of Sephadex G-25, washed with diluent buffer.
6. Elute with diluent buffer and collect fractions of 0.5 ml (approx.).
7. Measure fluorescence of each fraction in a 1 × 1 cm quartz cell using a 492 nm excitation filter and a 546 nm emission filter*.
8. The first peak contains the tracer, FITC-hPL; asses it as shown in Table 3.6.
9. Store tracer as deep-frozen aliquots.
10. The FIA assay is carried out as described in Table 1.3. The concentration of tracer has to be selected empirically, because current equipment is so variable. The aim should be a concentration at which the coefficient of variation of repeat determinations of fluorescence is of the order of $\leqslant 1\%$ (In the study on which this table was based (Chard and Sykes, 1979) the concentration was 0.5 μg/ml.) After separation of bound and free antigen fluorescence is measured either in the supernatant (free fraction) or in the precipitate after dissolving in 0.1 N NaOH (bound fraction).

---

* Current equipment, not being designed for FIA, varies considerably in its performance. Filters of the exact characteristics required may not be readily available, though provided they are within ± 5 nm of the desired wavelength will probably be adequate. Sensitivity can often be enhanced by the use of a 'broad pass' emission filter, i.e., which passes a total bandwidth of 10−20 nm around the optimum wavelength. At present a useful general purpose instrument for FIA is the Perkin-Elmer (models 1000 or 2000)

been described for γ-globulins (Tengerdy, 1965), albumin (Nargessi et al., 1978), gentamicin (Shaw, Watson and Smith, 1977), phenytoin (Kamel et al., 1978), placental lactogen (Chard and Sykes, 1979), α-fetoprotein (Sinosich and Chard, 1980), thyroxine and triiodothyronine (Curry et al., 1979), and insulin (Lidofsky et al., 1979). Fluorophores can also be used to label the antibody in systems comparable to the immunoradiometric assay (IRMA) (see § 6.4) and are referred to as 'immunofluorimetric

TABLE 4.6
Types of fluoroimmunoassay (FIA)

Type of assay	Heterogeneous (He) or Homogeneous (Ho)	Principle	Reference
Heterogeneous FIA	He	Fluorescent label replaces isotopic label on antigen	See text
Immunofluorometric assay (IFMA)	He or Ho	Fluorescent label replaces isotopic label on antibody	See text
Quenching FIA	Ho	Fluorescence quenched in bound fraction	Shaw et al., 1977
Fluorescent excitation transfer FIA	Ho	Fluorescent-labelled antigen and quencher-labelled antibody, fluorescence decreased in bound fraction	Ullman et al., 1976
Release FIA	Ho	Fluorophore released from tracer by enzymes	Burd et al., 1977
Enhancement FIA	Ho	Fluorescence enhanced in bound fraction	Smith, 1977
Indirect quenching FIA	Ho	Free fraction quenched with antisera to fluorescein	Nargessi et al., 1979

Polarisation FIA	Ho	Polarisation of emitted fluorescence increased in bound fraction	Dandliker et al., 1973; Watson et al., 1976; Kobayashi et al., 1979; Jolly et al., 1981
Fluorescence protection FIA	Ho	Fluorescent labelled antigen with antibodies to the antigen and fluorophore	Zuk et al., 1979
		Antibody to fluorophore quenches fluorescence of free but not bound fraction	—
Time-resolved FIA	Ho	Difference in fluorescent lifetimes between labelled antibody in free and bound phases	Richardson et al., 1979
Substrate-labelled FIA	Ho	Fluorogenic enzyme substrate is coupled to ligand. Fluorescence is released by enzyme hydrolysis in the free but not the bound fraction.	Wong et al., 1979

assay' (IFMA). IFMA procedures have been used for the quantitation of serum proteins using an antibody-coated stick and measurement of fluorescence on the surface of the stick (the FIAX/StiQ system) (Kameda et al., 1976). Similar procedures have been described using agarose beads as the support (Doelder and Ploem, 1974). Other immunofluorometric assays include those for pregnancy-specific β_1-glycoprotein (Sykes and Chard, 1980) and oestradiol (Ekeke et al., 1979). A method for a simple heterogeneous FIA is shown in Table 4.5.

Several ingenious systems of homogeneous fluoroimmunoassays have been described in which a separation step is unnecessary (Table 4.6).

4.4. Bacteriophage labels

A bacteriophage is a virus parasitic on bacteria; after replication it will destroy the host. This process is inhibited by antibodies to the bacteriophage itself or to antigens attached to the bacteriophage (Haimovich and Sela, 1966), and the phage can therefore act as the tracer in a binding assay. The first such system was an assay for angiotensin (Hurwitz et al., 1970). The antigen is covalently coupled to a bacteriophage; after incubation with antiserum and standards, the infective activity of the free phage was quantitated by translucent plaque formation (i.e., areas of destruction) on an agar plate layered with a culture of *Escherichia coli*. No separation procedure is necessary because the phage is inactive in the bound phase.

Systems of this type have not been widely employed because of the difficulties in preparing phage—antigen conjugates, the complexity of endpoint detection, and the likelihood of non-specific interference from biological samples.

4.5. Luminescent labels

Luminescence is associated with reactions which result in the emission of photons of light. The reaction may involve a synthetic chemical (chemiluminescence) such as the oxidation of luminol (5-amino-2,3'-dihydrophthalazine-1,4-dione) or acridinium compounds in the presence of H_2O_2

and a catalyst, or a biological reactant (bioluminescence) such as the luci-ferin–luciferase system. Using either of these as label, end-point detection could be exquisitely sensitive and, like fluorescence, very rapid. For ex-ample, the luciferin–luciferase system has been used to determine less than 10^{-13} M ATP (Hercules and Sheehan, 1978) and peroxidase-labelled an-tigen to determine nanogram quantities of staphylococcal enterotoxin B (Velan and Halmann, 1978). The luminescent material can be used for direct labelling of antigen or, in an interesting variation of the technique, a catalyst of the luminol reaction can act as the label – for example, the heme present in horseradish peroxidase covalently coupled to antibody (Olsson et al., 1979). However, technical difficulties have so far prevented the widespread application of luminescent labels in binding assays, not the least problem being the quenching of 99% or more of the luminescence after conjugation to biological materials. A luminescence immunoassay (LIA) for thyroxine has been described, but this depends on a complex column separation to remove interfering materials (Schroeder et al., 1979). For molecules circulating at high levels, such as IgG, relatively simple LIA procedures have been devised (Hersh et al., 1979).

4.6. Advantages of non-isotopic labels in binding assays

Isotopic labels continue to be used in the vast majority of current binding assays. Yet for many years it has been suggested that they will be rapidly overtaken by non-isotopic techniques. This is based on a number of po-tential advantages, and it is worthwhile to consider these in the light of the present stage of development of these procedures.

(1) *Radiation hazard*:   The elimination of the radiation hazard of iso-topes is, above all else, the principle reason for the development of alter-native labels. What is the nature of the hazard? Isotopes can be absorbed via a number of routes, including inhalation of volatile ^{125}I released into the atmosphere (see Appendix V). There is no doubt that performing a radioiodination with $\geqslant 1$ mCi of ^{125}I constitutes a risk which demands elaborate facilities and precautions. *However, most laboratories do not iodinate their own materials*. Actually performing a RIA involves at most a few μCi of ^{125}I; the amount of volatile ^{125}I released in the course of an

assay is $< 1\%$ of the total, and with simple precautions it is impossible for a technician to ingest or inhale more than a small fraction of the maximum permitted dose. Consumption of the entire tracer in a typical radioimmunoassay kit would cause no significant radiation effect — the dose is far less than that used in therapeutic ablation of the thyroid gland or even in many standard scanning procedures. This event might well prove lethal because of the content of preservatives such as sodium azide and so could apply equally to non-isotopic tracers.

Though it can be agreed that the radiation hazard of RIA is very small, this does not alter the fact that 'radioactivity' is an emotive subject which has led, in some parts of the world, to severe legislative restrictions on the use of isotopes. This may be a good, but not scientific reason for the development of alternative labels.

(2) *Stability of tracer*:   Isotopic tracers using ^{125}I are inherently unstable and have a useful shelf-life ranging from 3 weeks to 3 months. Some non-isotopic tracers have the great advantage of indefinite stability. For the typical laboratory user, accustomed to ordering even such immutable items as plastic tubes on a monthly cycle, this will have little impact. For the commercial manufacturer it has great merits, permitting preparation and quality control in bulk at widely spaced intervals, and making distribution a simple and comparatively leisurely procedure. This should, in turn, be reflected in price though it is interesting that, at the present time, kits based on non-isotopic labels are considerably more expensive than their isotopic counterparts.

(3) *End-point detection*:   Nothing could be easier or more precise than quantitation of radioactivity in a well-type γ-counter. Fluorescence may approach close to this ideal, but enzymes fall far short and demand attention to factors such as temperature and timing which grossly limit their practicality (Table 4.7). It has often been stated that the equipment for non-isotopic labels is simpler and cheaper than that for isotopes. This is totally false. Both EIA and FIA demand apparatus of a high level of sophistication which is invariably much more expensive than a simple manual γ-counter. Automation is an entirely separate issue.

(4) *Sensitivity*:   It has been claimed that the signal amplification available with labels such as enzymes and phages would much increase sensi-

TABLE 4.7

A comparison of end-point detection systems based on an arbitrary maximum score of 10

The values given are a subjective opinion (from Landon et al., 1979)

	Radioimmunoassay (γ-emitting isotope)	Radioimmunoassay (β-emitting isotope)	Enzymoimmunoassay	Fluoroimmunoassay
Precision	9	9	5	10
Sensitivity	10	10	Heterogeneous 10 Homogeneous 4	Heterogeneous 10 Homogeneous 4
Speed	8	4	5	10
Simplicity	9	2	5	10
Ability to check	10	10	2	10
Non-hazardous	2	2	10	10
Availability of instrumentation	9	5	10	5
Influence of biological samples	10	5	Heterogeneous 9 Homogeneous 5	Heterogeneous 9 Homogeneous 5

tivity. But it cannot be emphasised too strongly that isotope detection is *never* a limiting factor in the sensitivity of RIA, and that detection limits are dictated solely by binder affinity and assay design. In reality, many non-isotopic labels are relatively insensitive because of low signal-to-noise ratios.

(5) *Background noise*:   With the sole exception of samples from patients who have received radioactive isotopes, nothing can interfere with a radioactive signal. The same cannot be said for most alternative labels. Biological fluids invariably contain natural enzymes and fluorophores (e.g., bilirubin) and background noise is inevitable. For substances which circulate at high molar concentrations the level of tracer can be chosen so that this noise is relatively insignificant. With low concentrations and small amounts of tracer great care must be taken to eliminate background, involving, for example, the multiple wash steps in an ELISA system.

(6) *Separation procedures*:   Without any question, the single most important advantage of non-isotopic labels is the ability to design homogeneous systems which do not require separation of bound and free antigen. This is not feasible with isotopes. Elimination of the separation step greatly shortens and simplifies manual procedures, and has similar implications for the design of automated systems (see Ch. 13). Reducing the number of steps will improve precision, though this advantage may be lost again in the end-point detection. Furthermore, at the present time homogeneous systems only apply to small molecules, i.e. haptens.

(7) *Automation*:   It is noted elsewhere (Ch. 13) that the major stumbling block to the automation of binding assays is the separation procedure. If this is eliminated then the design of appropriate systems becomes relatively straightforward. This is another important potential benefit of homogeneous non-isotopic immunoassays.

4.7. Conclusions – the place of non-isotopic binding assays

Generalisations are not easy in this fast-moving subject, and any conclusions may be overtaken by the present rapid developments in non-iso-

TABLE 4.8

Approximate circulating levels, in molar terms, of a variety of natural substances (from Landon et al., 1979)

Substance	mmol/l	Substance	µmol/l	Substance	nmol/l	Substance	pmol/l
Sodium	140	Albumin	600	Oestriol (late pregnancy)	600	Aldosterone	180
Chloride	105	Urate	250	Thyroxine-binding globulin	500	Insulin	120
Bicarbonate	30	Phenylalanine	125	Cortisol	400	Parathyroid hormone	100
Glucose	5	Immunoglobulin G	90	Placental lactogen	300	Growth hormone	50
Urea	4	Ammonia	30	Thyroxine (total)	125	Luteinising hormone	10
Cholesterol	4	Iron	20	Corticosterone	20	Triiodothyronine (free)	10
Calcium	2.5	Bilirubin (total)	10	Triiodothyronine	2	Adrenocorticotrophin	10
Triglycerides (fasting)	1	Immunoglobulin M	1	Prolactin	1	Thyroid stimulating hormone	5
				Oestradiol 17β (women)	1	Angiotensin 11	4
				Progesterone	1	Oxytocin	1

topic immunoassay. Furthermore, there is a tendency to think of this whole group of techniques in terms of EIA, whereas the major future advances probably lie in fluorescence and luminescence. Nevertheless, the following conclusions may be put forward based on the current state of the art:

(1) Only heterogeneous EIA can match the sensitivity of RIA for substances whose levels are in pmol/l or nmol/l (Table 4.8); these procedures are cumbersome and imprecise and unlikely, therefore, to replace RIA;

(2) Homogeneous EIA and FIA can be applied to many substances whose levels are in the high nmol/l or μmol/l; if precision is adequate, they are valid alternatives to RIA;

(3) Both heterogeneous and homogeneous EIA and FIA should be suitable for materials which circulate at relatively high levels, and where the desired result is a 'yes' or a 'no' rather than precise quantitation; examples include screening for antibodies to infectious diseases, detection of hepatitis-associated antigen, and detection of chorionic gonadotrophin as an early pregnancy test;

(4) Non-isotopic assays must be the method of choice in situations in which there are severe legislative restrictions on RIA.

CHAPTER 5

Requirements for binding assays – the binder

The characteristics of a radioimmunoassay or similar technique will depend above all on the properties of the binder. Of the available binders, specific antibodies are much the most widely used – in combination with an isotopic tracer, as a radioimmunoassay. Less widely used, though still of importance, are assays based on naturally occurring circulating binders (commonly referred to as 'competitive protein binding assays') or cellular receptors ('receptor assays'). Finally, there is a small group of less familiar methods which employ the same basic principle but are not commonly thought of as binder assays, for example the use of an enzyme as 'binder' for its substrate, providing a means for measuring that substrate.

5.1. Antibodies and the immune response

5.1.1. Chemistry of antibodies

Antibody molecules or 'immunoglobulins' are found in the slower running fractions of serum proteins on electrophoresis – among the β and γ globulins. The 'immunoglobulins' comprise five distinct classes, referred to as IgG, IgM, IgA, IgD and IgE, all based on a common underlying structure (see Fig. 5.1). Each class has a characteristic spectrum of activity: for example, the IgE class contains the 'reagins', which are responsible for allergic phenomena such as asthma. The IgM class is the major immunoglobulin of several primitive species; in higher animals the earliest phase of the immune response includes IgM antibodies which subsequently disappear, an example of ontogeny repeating phylogeny. However, from the point of view of radioimmunoassay only one class is of any significance, IgG, since the latter includes the vast majority of the anti-

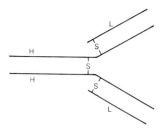

Fig. 5.1. The structure of the IgG molecule, consisting of two heavy chains (H) and two light chains (L) linked by disulphide bridges (S).

bodies arising from specific artificial immunisation. The IgG class also includes most of the familiar antibodies to bacterial and viral antigens, and thus plays an important role in the body's defence mechanisms.

IgG consists of four peptide chains linked by disulphide bonds, (Fig. 5.1): two so-called 'heavy' or H chains and two 'light' or L chains. The whole molecule is ~160,000 M_r. Immunoglobulins of other classes have the same basic structure but differ:

(1) In the amino acid sequence of the constant portion of the H chain;

(2) In their tendency to form polymers.

IgM for example, consists of 5 basic units linked in a ring structure. The M_r differences, expressed as the sedimentation coefficient in an ultracentrifuge, formed the basis of an earlier terminology for immunoglobulins which divide them into two groups: 7 S (mostly IgG); and 19 S (IgM).

The functional activity of the different parts of the IgG molecule was originally defined on the basis of experiments in which purified IgG was subjected to limited enzyme digestion (Porter, 1959). Papain splits IgG into three fragments (Fig. 5.2). Two of these are identical and consist of a light chain and the adjacent part of the heavy chain; this is the Fab fragment, so-called because it contains the combining site of the molecule. The third fragment consists of the remaining parts of the heavy chains; this is the Fc fragment, so-called because it can be crystallised. The Fc fragment, which also includes the carbohydrate moiety of the IgG molecule, is responsible for secondary activities such as the fixation of complement. IgG can also be split by pepsin, yielding two fragments: one is

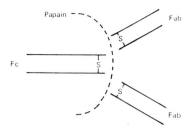

Fig. 5.2. Cleavage of the IgG molecule by the enzyme papain yielding two Fab fragments, each containing one antibody combining site, and one Fc fragment.

Fc; the other is equivalent to two Fab fragments and is referred to as $F(ab')_2$.

The N-terminal half of the Fab piece shows great variability, and is thus referred to as the 'variable' or V region. The C-terminal half is relatively constant, and referred to as the 'constant' or C region. The combining site lies in the variable region, and it is this variability, with the potential existence of many millions of different structures, which is responsible for the great specificity of antibodies. It is also, in part, responsible for the heterogeneity of an antibody population directed to a single antigen. In the course of the immune response large numbers of antibody molecules are produced with slightly different variable regions. Some fit the antigen very closely and thus have a high affinity; others with a less close fit are of lower affinity.

5.1.2. Chemistry of antigens

Most substances of $M_r \geqslant 300$ can stimulate an immune response with the formation of specific antibodies. Up to M_r 1,000 the antigen must be coupled to a larger molecule in order to be immunogenic; above this M_r-value most materials are immunogenic on their own.

The antibody-combining site corresponds in size to approximately 4 amino acids or 6 hexoses (Goodman, 1975), or to a typical steroid molecule (Kuss et al., 1978). Studies by X-ray crystallography have shown that the binding site may take the form of a shallow groove (15 Å x 6 Å x 6 Å), a wedge-shaped cavity (12 Å x 15 Å x 20 Å), or a conical cavity (10 Å diam.) (Blake, 1975). In the case of proteins it would appear that the antigenic site is usually conformational rather than sequential (Sela, 1969); in other words, the site is not a single sequence of amino acids but rather one or more amino acids in different parts of the peptide chain which happen to be juxtaposed because of the tertiary structure of the molecule. This has been confirmed by Atassi (1978) who has defined the antigenic structure of egg-white lysozyme as including six amino acid residues which are closely related in the three-dimensional structure but distant in sequence. A synthetic peptide containing these amino acids alone had immunochemical properties similar to those of the whole lysozyme molecule, thus opening exciting possibilities for synthetic immunogens and tracers.

5.1.3. Cellular basis of the immune response

The basic cells involved in the immune response are small lymphocytes derived from the bone marrow known as 'B' lymphocytes. These cells carry on their surface IgG molecules similar to those which they secrete when stimulated, a type of biological 'free sample'. The mechanisms by which individual cells secrete molecules of a single specificity is not at present clear. Two theories have been put forward:

(1) The 'germ-line theory', suggesting that the genes for all types of variable region are present in every cell, but that in a given cell only one gene is expressed;

(2) The 'somatic mutation theory' suggests that the variability is generated within the individual cell by a series of mutations.

But whatever the underlying mechanism, it now seems certain that the surface receptors determine those cells which will be stimulated, and thus the specificity of the antibody response. Lymphocytes of the B series are found in a variety of sites, including the marrow, spleen, lymph glands and blood.

With the exception of some large antigens of regular structure such as polysaccharides, most substances require some sort of processing before they can efficiently stimulate the B lymphocytes. One such system is provided by macrophages which take up the antigen at the site of injection; the antigen is then released, possibly as a complex with RNA, in a form which can directly stimulate the B lymphocyte. Another system may be operative in the case of 'haptens': these are small M_r materials such as steroid hormones which can bind to antibody, but cannot themselves stimulate the immune response unless linked to a larger 'carrier' molecule such as a protein. The carrier is recognised by and stimulates another class of lymphocytes derived from the thymus and variously known as 'T' lymphocytes or 'helper T cells'. These, in turn, stimulate the B cells; the histocompatibility antigens of the B and T cells are a key factor in this process. A further factor which may stimulate the B lymphocytes is complement, and this can be activated by some antigens.

The bulk of antibody produced is secreted by plasma cells. These are derived from small lymphocytes as a result of antigenic stimulation, and differ from them in having more cytoplasm and an abundant endoplasmic reticulum (i.e., they have the appropriate machinery for protein synthesis and export).

5.1.4. Physiology of the immune response

Classically the immune response is divided into primary and secondary phases. The primary response follows the first administration of antigen; although only small amounts of antibody are then produced, it is the phase during which the small population of specifically-programmed lymphocytes differentiate and proliferate to form a much larger population. The secondary response follows the second or subsequent administration of antigen; acting on the now much larger population of programmed lymphocytes, it results in the production of large quantities of antibody. The number of cells capable of responding is probably the underlying basis of the 'memory' which characterises immune responses in general; this is the greatly enhanced reaction to a second or subsequent exposure to the antigen.

In practice, the distinction between the primary and secondary response may be blurred by the nature of the immunisation process. For the production of antisera, the antigen is usually injected with an adjuvant (see § 5.2.4), one action of which is to slow the release of antigen from the injection site. If this process is sufficiently prolonged, then the response will pass from the primary to the secondary phase following a single administration.

At one time it was believed that an animal could not mount an immune response to its own antigens: the phenomenon of 'self-recognition'. However, there are now numerous instances of successful immunisation with materials which occur naturally in the animal. Examples include the steroid hormones, and the posterior pituitary peptides, which have the same chemical structure in a variety of species. The presence of circulating antibody to an endogenous hormone can have striking effects: thus animals immunised against vasopressin (the antidiuretic hormone) will occasionally develop diabetes insipidus with severe polyuria and polydipsia; animals immunised against sex steroids can exhibit alterations in gonadal function (see Nieschlag, 1975).

5.2. Preparation of antisera for use in RIA

5.2.1. Production of antibodies

A typical immunisation schedule is shown in Table 5.1. The details are somewhat arbitrary, since there must be almost as many different approaches as there are workers in the field of immunoassay. In practice, it is difficult to show that any one scheme is better than any other, because of the very variable nature of the antibody response. Claims for a particular method are usually based on anecdotes which cannot be reproduced in the hands of other workers.

Despite the uncertainties, there are certain specific factors which can be discussed in relation to the success or otherwise of an immunisation procedure. These are:
(1) The nature of the immunogen and its dose;
(2) The adjuvant;
(3) The animal species used; the route of immunisation;
(4) The timing of injection and collection of antisera.

5.2.2. The nature and dose of the immunogen

In general, the immunogenicity*, of a material is directly related to its

---

* Immunogen must be distinguished from 'antigen'. An immunogen is material which will stimulate an immune response; an antigen is a material which will react with an antibody, but is not necessarily immunogenic on its own (e.g., most haptens)

TABLE 5.1

An immunisation schedule

Production of antiserum to human placental lactogen (hPL)

1. Dissolve 0.6 mg of purified hPL in 2 ml phosphate buffer (Table 1.4) containing no protein (use a glass tube).
2. Add 4.5 ml of complete Freund's adjuvant (Difco).
3. Homogenise thoroughly: A convenient method for this is repeated aspiration and expulsion from an all-glass syringe fitted with an all-metal needle. Plastic should be avoided as some types are attacked by components of the adjuvant. An alternative method is the use of a Potter-Elvehjem homogeniser.
4. Inject 1 ml of the homogenate into each of 6 adult female New Zealand White rabbits. The injection should be subcutaneous and divided among 6 or more sites around the neck and shoulders. There is no need to shave the animal for this procedure.
5. Wait 6 weeks and repeat the procedure, but using 25 μg immunogen/animal rather than 100 μg.
6. After a further 2 weeks take a test bleed (2 ml) and repeat the booster immunisation when this has been examined.
7. Repeat for 4 booster injections in total, and then repeat at 1–3 month intervals according to the results and the requirements for antiserum.
8. If the test bleed reveals a useful antiserum, a larger bleed (50 ml) should be collected prior to the next booster injection.
9. For a larger animal (sheep, goat) a similar schedule may be followed but the amount of immunogen should be increased 2–3 times.

Note: If, with an 'easy' immunogen, an animal has shown either no response or a poor response by the second test bleed then it should be eliminated from the series

M_r-value. Materials of $> 5,000$ M_r are usually good immunogens; for example, if hPL (M_r 20,000) is injected with adjuvant into a group of 6 rabbits, most will respond and at least 2 are likely to produce appropriate antisera. However, 'appropriate' must be related to the actual demands of the assay; if very high sensitivity is required and thus antisera of exceptionally high affinity, the success rate may be considerably less. By contrast, the immune response to small peptides such as ACTH (M_r 4,500) and the posterior pituitary hormones (M_r 1,000) is often poor or non-existent, and large numbers of animals may have to be injected and tested before an efficient antiserum is found. Conjugation of small peptides to proteins, or absorption to carbon particles (Boyd et al., 1968), is of doubtful value. Materials of $< 800 \, M_r$ are non-immunogenic, but may become so when conjugated, as 'hapten', to a larger molecule such as albumin (see § 5.2.3).

There is no simple dose—response relationship in the immune response and the amount of immunogen is non-critical over a wide range. Most workers use doses of 50—100 μg, though much smaller amounts may be effective. This is illustrated by the common occurrence of 'non-specific' antibodies to contaminants which represent 10% or less of the preparation used for immunisation. At the other end of the scale, doses of 1 mg or more may produce the phenomenon of 'tolerance' in the recipient animal, with no response to either this or subsequent injections of the immunogen.

It is often stated that less pure material is more immunogenic than highly purified material. But the evidence for this is anecdotal and of doubtful validity. As a general rule, and where sufficient quantities are available, the most highly purified material should be used for immunisation. This is particularly the case with materials prepared synthetically, since they may include contaminants closely related to the pure antigen.

If the immunogen is identical or closely related to endogenous material in the recipient animal, the antibodies which result may react with the material both at the site of origin and in the circulation. This may alter the apparent characteristics of the antiserum. Endogenous antigen will bind to the antibodies of highest affinity; if the dissociation constant is low, the process is effectively irreversible and the antiserum will appear to be of relatively low affinity. In situations where this may occur, it is worthwhile to test the antiserum before and after treatment designed to split the antigen—antibody complex (e.g., with acid or chaotropic agents such as urea), and to separate free antigen and antibody (e.g., by dialysis or gel filtration).

5.2.3. Preparation of haptens as immunogens

The carriers most widely used for preparing small molecules as immunogens are proteins such as albumin, thyroglobulin and keyhole limpet haemocyanin; a case can also be made for the use of purified histocompatibility antigens which may be an essential part of the immune response (see § 5.1.3). A covalent link has to be formed between the proteins and the hapten, usually a peptide bond between a carboxyl on the small molecule and a free amino group on the protein molecule (the sidechain of lysine residues). If the small molecule does not have a carboxyl group then a derivative must be formed (Table 5.2). The derivatives also serve the purpose of providing a 'bridge' of 4–6 carbon atoms between the haptens and the carrier; this improves specificity by ensuring that the hapten projects above the hydrated surface of the protein. Methods of forming hapten–protein links are described in Appendix VI (see also Erlanger, 1973).

The number of hapten molecules which can attach to a protein molecule depends on the number of free amino groups in the latter. For albumin the number is 60. A minimum number of sites must be occupied for the immunogen to be effective (15–30 in the case of albumin). Oversubstitution may be counter-productive. The use of thyroglobulin, which presents at least 400 sites, has been advocated.

The site of linkage between the hapten and the protein is of critical importance for the specificity of the antiserum. The most distinctive groups of the hapten should be remote from the linkage site and thus presented to the immune system of the animal in unaltered form. For example, with an oestrogen the site should not be on the highly charac-

TABLE 5.2

Examples of derivatives through which a small molecule which does not possess an amino or a carboxyl group may be conjugated to amino-groups of proteins (see Erlanger (1973) for principles and methods of making hapten–protein conjugates)

Active group on small molecule	Carboxyl-containing derivative
Ketone	Carboxymethyl oxime
Hydroxyl	Succinate
	Glutarate
	Chlorocarbonate
Phenol	P-Aminobenzoate

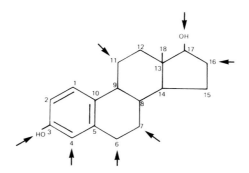

Fig. 5.3. The oestradiol molecule showing the sites through which it can be conjugated to a protein molecule in the preparation of an immunogen. Conjugates through the 6 position are much favoured because they leave exposed most of the characteristic sites of the molecule.

teristic A ring (see Fig. 5.3). The most specific antisera to oestrogens have been those raised against conjugates through the C-6 or C-7 position; for progesterone the C-11 position is favoured, and for cortisol C-3.

Not all hapten–protein conjugates are equally successful as immunogens and whether or not specificity can be achieved between two closely related molecules may depend on the exact position at which the difference occurs. With steroid hormones, for example, the C-17 position is 'sterically unhindered' and it is possible to raise antisera which distinguish almost completely between 17-hydroxyl and 17-keto compounds. By contrast, the 11-position is 'sterically hindered' by the adjacent C-18 and C-19 methyl groups, and most antisera cannot distinguish between different substituents at this site (see Pratt, 1978). Similarly, specific antisera to prostaglandins of the A and F groups have proved relatively easy to produce, while those for the E groups have given rise to considerable problems.

5.2.4. The use of adjuvant

In most immunisation schedules the antigen is injected as an emulsion in 'complete Freund's adjuvant'. This is a mixture of mineral oil, detergent, and killed mycobacteria (adjuvant without the latter is referred to as 'incomplete'). The mineral oil, being hydrophobic, tends to remain at the site of the injection and thus to delay absorption; the droplets are slowly removed by the macrophages of the reticuloendothelial system, and the contained antigen is thus progressively released by a route which will provide maximal exposure to the immune system. The detergent serves as an emulsifying agent, so that the aqueous solution of antigen is contained within the droplets of mineral oil (Fig. 5.4). In order to ensure a 'water-in-oil' rather than an 'oil-in-water' emulsion, the proportion of adjuvant to antigen solution should always be 2 : 1 (v/v) or greater and the resulting emulsion should be tested by dispersion on a water surface. The killed mycobacteria provide a non-specific stimulus to the reticuloendothelial and immune systems with proliferation of macrophages and lymphocytes both locally and systemically. Some workers have employed pre-treatment with *Bordetella pertussis* antigen in order to achieve this effect.

5.2.5 The animal species

Consistent differences between species in their response to a given immunogen have rarely been shown. Inbred strains may occasionally show a difference; for example, one strain of guinea pig will not respond to DNP (Green et al., 1969). However, this is an exception rather than the rule, and the choice of animal is usually determined by the facilities available. Other things being equal, a large species such as the goat or the sheep would be chosen; if an efficient antiserum is obtained, it is then available in substantial quantities (1 litre or more). Laboratories which

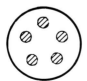   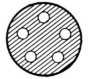

'Water-in-oil' emulsion   'Oil-in-water' emulsion

Fig. 5.4. The two types of emulsion which can be formed when a solution of an immunogen is homogenised in complete Freund's adjuvant. A water-in-oil emulsion is desirable and can be achieved by using a relative excess of the adjuvant by volume.

do not have access to accommodation for larger animals will usually use rabbits or guinea pigs. With some antisera of high titre and affinity, small volumes may suffice for immense numbers of assays, and quantity is not invariably a major criterion.

5.2.6. The route of immunisation

The immune response is systemic rather than local, and this may explain why the results of immunisation by different routes are very similar. Nevertheless, a number of different injection sites have been advocated (Table 5.3).

5.2.7. The timing of injections and collection of antisera

Because variation is so great all that can be offered are simple rules of thumb for the timing of injection. The protocol shown in Table 5.1 is known to work, but shorter or longer intervals might be equally effective. To explore the question would require more work than is usually devoted to the development of a complete radioimmunoassay system, and the results would apply only to the particular immunogen studied.

TABLE 5.3
Routes of injection for immunisation

Route	Comments
Intradermal	Multiple (40+) small (~25 μl) injections over a wide area of body surface (Vaitukaitis et al., 1971). Rapid response after a single immunisation
Subcutaneous	The most widely used method (Table 5.1)
Intramuscular	Rarely used
Intraperitoneal	Rarely used
Intravenous	Rarely used, only applicable without adjuvant
Intranodal	Direct injection into lymph-nodes (Boyd et al., 1967). Very tedious and no better than other routes
Footpad	Extremely painful for animal, should never be used

Antiserum is usually collected 1 or 2 weeks after a booster injection
(a 'typical' response is shown in Fig. 5.5). In some animals the titre is
maintained for months or years in the absence of further booster injections; in others it shows a progressive fall.

5.2.8. Selection of antisera for use in a radioimmunoassay

An immunisation programme will yield a number of antisera from which
one or more must be selected for use in an assay. The criteria for this
selection are specificity, affinity and titre.

(1) *Specificity*:   This must be the primary criterion; unless an antiserum has the appropriate specificity it will be of no value in the assay
regardless of its affinity and titre.

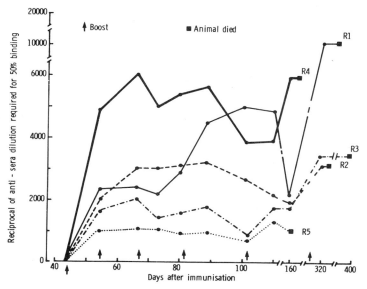

Fig. 5.5. Immunisation of 5 rabbits (R1–5) with a conjugate of oestriol (E_3) to
bovine serum albumin. Each booster injection is shown by an arrow, and the titre is
expressed as the reciprocal of the antiserum dilution required to bind 50% of a
tracer of $[^3H]E_3$. Note the striking increase in titre after the first booster injection,
but the very variable response thereafter.

(2) *Affinity*:   Sensitivity of an assay is closely related to the affinity or
K-value of the antibody (see § 1.7) and in general the antiserum of highest
K-value, as indicated by a Scatchard plot, will be selected for use. Heterogeneity of apparent K-value, as reflected by a Scatchard plot which yields
a curve rather than a straight line, may also be an important factor as it
will tend to reduce the slope of the standard curve (Fig. 5.6).

(3) *Titre*:   Given antisera of equivalent specificity and affinity, the titre
(expressed as the reciprocal of the dilution which will bind 50% of a
tracer) may determine the final choice. Thus an antiserum with a titre
of 1 : 50,000 would be preferred to one with a titre of 1 : 20,000 because
it would yield more assay tubes per ml of the raw serum. It should be
emphasised that titre does not directly reflect affinity since it is also a
function of the total antibody concentration. Two different antisera
would yield identical dilution curves if the one contained 10-times as
much antibody of 1/10th of the K-value of the other.

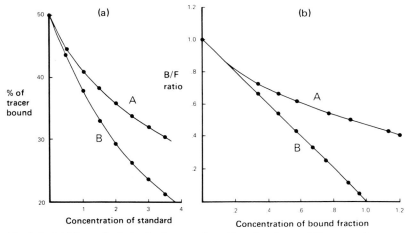

Fig. 5.6.   (a) Theoretical standard curves for a ligand and two different antisera to
that ligand. (b) Scatchard plots derived from the standard curves of (a). Antiserum
B contains a single population of antibodies with a single K-value and therefore
yields a straight line on the Scatchard plot. Antiserum A contains multiple populations of antibodies of different K-value and yields a curve on the Scatchard plot.
If the aim of the assay is to yield the best possible dynamic range over concentrations of 0–4 then clearly antibody B is much the best.

5.2.9. Storage of antisera

Serum is preferable to plasma because it is less likely to form cryoprecipitates. The serum should be divided into aliquots and stored at $-20°C$ to minimise the potential damaging effects of repeated freezing and thawing. The size of each aliquot will depend both on the total volume and on the rate at which the antiserum is used; in general a thawed aliquot stored at $2-4°C$ with a preservative such as 0.1% sodium azide will be stable for at least 3–6 months.

5.3. Monoclonal antibodies

A recent development with important implications for immunoassay is the production of so-called 'monoclonal' antibodies (Kohler and Milstein, 1976; Milstein and Kohler, 1977). Antibody-producing cells are harvested from an immunised animal and incubated in vitro with a line of mouse myeloma cells known to grow efficiently in tissue culture. Under appropriate conditions some of the antibody-producing cells fuse or 'hybridise' with the myeloma cells, and the result is a cell line producing both the myeloma immunoglobulins, *and* the antibody immunoglobulin of the immunised animal. In other words, the ability to produce the antibody is transferred from cells which will not normally thrive in culture to cells which will thrive, and which can therefore produce the antibody indefinitely and on any scale, either in vitro, or in vivo by re-injection into the peritoneal cavity of an intact animal.

It is then possible to select from among the fused cells those which are producing antibody of the desired characteristics, and to grow these cells as 'clones'. A given clone should produce a single species of antibody immunoglobulin, hence the term 'monoclonal' antibodies.

The potential advantages of monoclonal antibody systems are:
(1) Once a clone has been established, it can produce antibodies indefinitely. Furthermore, the cells can be stored or distributed, so that one clone could in principle supply the entire world demand for a given antibody forever.
(2) At the cloning stage it is possible to select cells producing 'perfect' antibody, even if these represent only a small fraction of the total population.

(3) The resulting antibody is a pure, single species of immunoglobulin. It should, therefore, lend itself extremely well to the attractive immunometric systems (see § 6.4), one of the main problems of which is to purify antibodies from a heterogeneous population of immunoglobulins. Much preliminary data on the use of monoclonal antibodies in RIA suggested that affinity, and hence sensitivity, would be relatively low. However, practical systems have now been described for materials circulating in the pmol/l range (e.g., hGH, Bundesen et al., 1980; AFP, Votila et al., 1981; progesterone, Eshhar et al., 1981).

5.4. Cell receptors

The first step in the action of any hormone involves binding to a specific receptor which then activates the cellular machinery for the hormonal response. The receptors for steroid hormones reside in the target cell cytoplasm, for thyroid hormones in the nucleus, and for protein hormones on the cell surface membrane. The use of isolated cell receptors as the binding agent in an assay has one great advantage – that it should measure the functional site of the molecule. Other binders, by contrast, may associate with parts of the molecule remote from the functional site and thus measure inactive fragments. Cell receptors also have high affinity constants and therefore have the potential for yielding a very sensitive assay (e.g., 1–10 pg for corticotrophin). For these reasons the concept of receptor assays has been enthusiastically received within recent years. The first such assay to be described was that for oestrogens using the uterine cytosol receptor (Korenman, 1968). Subsequently, procedures have been described for a variety of materials including corticotrophin (Lefkowitz et al., 1970), gonadotrophins employing cell-surface receptors extracted from the appropriate target organs (Catt et al., 1972), cyclic AMP using a binding protein from skeletal muscle (Gilman, 1970) and neuroleptic drugs using extracts of rat brain (Creese and Synder, 1977).

Receptor assays have a number of disadvantages:

(1) Their functional specificity may embrace molecules which are chemically very different: for example, the long-acting thyroid stimulator (LATS) can cross-react in a radioreceptor assay for TSH (Mehdi, 1975).

(2) A substantial proportion of cell-surface receptors may not be involved in the biological response of the cell and their functional specificity is therefore in doubt (Birnbaumer and Pohl, 1973).

(3) Receptor assays are only applicable to those materials for which recognisable receptors exist; they cannot be used for substances such as α-fetoprotein or coagulation factors which have no function in the hormonal sense.

(4) More importantly, receptor assays are seriously limited in their practicality. The preparation of the receptor involves homogenisation of tissue and fractionation of the extract by ultracentrifugation; with a complex procedure of this type considerable batch-to-batch variation may occur. Furthermore, because many receptor preparations are unstable, new batches have to be prepared at frequent intervals. The requirements for the purity of the tracer are also much more stringent than those which apply to a radioimmunoassay.

These practical considerations explain why receptor assays have not yet found much application outside research units, though a receptor assay for chorionic gonadotrophin (hCG) is widely used in clinical practice (Landesman and Saxena, 1976).

Radioreceptor assays may have a special and unique place in the definition of systems in which several chemically different molecules have a similar biological effect. For example, the radioreceptor assays for insulin, using isolated fat cells of liver membranes as the binder, react not only to insulin but also to the so-called 'non-suppressible, insulin-like activity' (NSILA) which is probably one of the somatomedins (Van Wyk et al., 1974). Recognition of the presence of opiate receptors in the mammalian brain led to the development of assays which permitted identification of the endorphins and enkephalins. Another application of increasing importance is direct measurement of the receptors themselves, illustrated by the determination of oestrogen receptors in breast cancer (see § 5.6), and the demonstration that insulin resistance in certain patients may be due to a deficiency of insulin receptors rather than the presence of endogenous antibodies to insulin (Soll et al., 1975).

5.5. Circulating binding proteins

The steroid and thyroid hormones are associated in the circulation with specific binding proteins: cortisol binding globulin (CBG) for the corticosteroids and progesterone; sex hormone binding globulin (SHBG) for oestrogens and androgens; and thyroxine binding globulin (TBG) for thyroxine and triiodothyronine. Because of the presence of these proteins the bulk of the active compound in blood is in the form of a bound complex, leaving a small free fraction which is responsible for biological activity. Natural binders also exist for the haematinics, folate and B12.

The circulating binding proteins have been widely used as the binder in assays for the relevant ligand, and have the advantage that the primary material is reproducible and widely available. The usual source is serum from women in late pregnancy which contains high levels of all the binding proteins; folate is assayed with a binding protein from milk, and vitamin B12 with extracts of gastric mucosa (intrinsic factor) or serum from the toadfish (Kubiatowicz et al., 1977). However, this type of assay has several important disadvantages:

(1) The binding proteins have relatively low affinity constants ($10^7 - 10^8$ ℓ/mol when compared with antibodies and thus cannot yield a very sensitive assay;

(2) Their specificity is poor — for example, SHBG will bind a wide range of oestrogens and 17-hydroxyandrogens and the measurement of any one of these requires preliminary extraction and purification; the vitamin B12-binding proteins obtained from gastric mucosa include both intrinsic factor (which binds B12 specifically), and the so-called 'R-protein' which binds a variety of B12 analogues; assays in which the binder contains 'R-protein' can fail to diagnose a B12 deficiency state (Kolhouse et al., 1978);

(3) The affinity constant is very temperature-dependent and the assays have to be conducted under carefully controlled low temperatures;

(4) Because of the low affinity constant, the binder has to be used at high concentration and therefore demands the collection of large pools of primary material; with an antiserum by contrast, the product of one animal may be sufficient for many millions of assays.

For these reasons most assays depending on a circulating binding protein have been replaced by radioimmunoassays. The only notable exceptions are vitamin D, folate, and vitamin B12, and in the latter case an antibody has been described (Endres et al., 1978).

5.6. Radioassay for the detection of endogenous antibodies, circulating binding proteins and receptors

Principles similar to that of radioimmunoassay can be applied to the measurement of endogenous binder in the sample. Examples include:

(1) *Sex hormone-binding globulin*: The SHBG binding sites are saturated with 5-α-[^{3}H]dihydrotestosterone. SHBG is then selectively precipitated with ammonium sulphate, and the amount of [^{3}H]DHT bound gives a direct measurement of SHBG concentration (Rosner, 1972). Here, DHT is used as ligand in preference to testosterone because it has a higher affinity for SHBG.

(2) *Thyroxine-binding globulin*: Binding sites on TBG not occupied by thyroxine (T_4) are saturated with [^{125}I]triidothyronine (T_3). Bound and free T_3 are then separated by one of a variety of methods of which the most familiar depend on adsorption of the free T_3 to a resin (Mitchell et al., 1960). In this case the tracer (T_3) has a lower affinity for the binding protein than the endogenous ligand (T_4). Thus the result is determined by both the total TBG *and* the total T_4 present and the test is frequently combined with a direct assay of T_4 to yield a 'free thyroxine index'. The procedure is widely used in the assessment of thyroid function and goes under a variety of names including 'thyroid hormone uptake test' or 'THUT', and 'T_3 resin uptake'. It should be noted that direct assays of TBG in blood are becoming increasingly popular (Levy et al., 1971; Hesch et al., 1976), and that, together with simpler methods for the measurement of 'free' T_4 (Odstrchel et al., 1978), may replace the classical T_3 uptake methods.

(3) *Antibodies to growth hormone (hGH)*: Dwarf children on long-term treatment with purified growth hormone frequently develop antibodies to this material. These can be quantitated by binding studies using a tracer of ^{125}I-labelled hGH, serial dilutions of the patient's serum,

and separation of bound and free hGH by second antibody specific to human immunoglobulins (see § 6.3.5.1).

(4) *Specific IgE antibodies*:   Allergic disorders (e.g., hay-fever, asthma) are associated with the presence of endogenous antibodies of the IgE class (see § 5.1.1) specific to one or more of a variety of allergens. The patient's serum is reacted with solid phase allergen which binds allergen-specific IgE antibodies. The solid-phase is then reacted with labelled anti-IgE antibodies; the amount of radioactivity bound is directly related to the amount of allergen-specific IgE in the sample. This is the so-called 'radio-allergosorbent test' or 'RAST' (Wide et al., 1967).

(5) *Oestrogen receptors in breast cancer*:   Normal breast tissue contains oestrogen receptors (ER). Neoplastic tissue may or may not contain ER, and on this finding depends the use of therapeutic endocrine manipulations (McGuire, 1973). Cell cytosol from tissue extracts is incubated with tritiated oestradiol ($[^3H]E_2$) in series of tubes containing graded amounts of non-radioactive E_2. Unbound $[^3H]E_2$ is adsorbed to charcoal to determine the distribution of bound and free, and the results assessed by Scatchard plot analysis to give the concentration of binder present (see § 1.6).

(6) *Insulin receptors*:   A direct radioassay for insulin receptors has been described based on the use of ^{125}I-labelled purified receptor, and an endogenous antibody to the receptor found in the serum of some patients with insulin-resistant diabetes (Harrison et al., 1979).

CHAPTER 6

Requirements for binding assays – separation of bound and free ligand

Once the primary binder–ligand reaction is complete it is necessary to determine the distribution of the ligand between the free and the bound form. Usually, but not always, this requires that the bound fraction be physically separated from the free fraction, and a variety of techniques have been described for this purpose. All such techniques exploit physicochemical differences between the ligand in its free and bound forms: for example, the addition of an organic solvent at a concentration which will precipitate binder molecules and thus a binder–ligand complex, but which will not precipitate the unbound ligand.

The main operative criteria for a separation procedure are efficiency and practicality. These will be considered in turn, followed by a discussion of the currently available methods.

6.1. Efficiency of separation procedures

The efficiency of a separation procedure can be defined as the completeness with which the bound and free phases are separated (Fig. 6.1). It is worthwhile to examine the meaning of this definition and to consider the relative contributions to overall efficiency made by the separation procedure on the one hand and by the primary reagents on the other.

In theory, a perfect separation system would completely divide the two components of the assay. In practice this is never achieved for two reasons:

(1) *Free ligand behaves as 'bound'*: It is always found that a fraction of the free ligand behaves identically with the bound, and does so even in the absence of the binder: this is variously referred to as the 'diluent' or

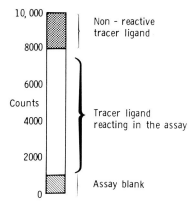

Fig. 6.1. Diagrammatic illustration of the efficiency of a separation procedure. In a perfect assay all of the tracer ligand would distribute between the bound and free phases. In practice, some of the free will be classified as bound (assay blank) and some of the bound as the free (non-reactive tracer). This arises because most tracers contain impurities, and because no separation procedure is completely efficient in the separation of bound and free ligand. The properties shown here would vary considerably between different ligands and different separation procedures.

'assay blank', or 'non-specific binding', or as 'misclassification error'. For example, a procedure which uses a chemical precipitation of the bound complex can invariably be shown to precipitate a proportion of the free ligand in control tubes containing no binder and this holds even when the ligand should be completely soluble under the conditions chosen. There are several possible explanations of this phenomenon:

(i) Physical trapping of free ligand in the bound complex, for instance in the interstices of a precipitate; this phenomenon can be quantitated by observing the effect of repeated washing of the precipitate, or following the distribution of an isotope such as ^{22}Na which appears solely in the liquid phase;

(ii) The presence in the tracer ligand of impurities with chemical properties similar to those of the bound complex;

(iii) Absorption of free ligand, for instance to the walls of the assay tube;

(iv) Incomplete separation of the two phases because the relevant properties of the free ligand are similar to though not identical with those of the bound complex (see Fig. 6.6).

In practical terms it is often difficult to identify the process responsible for the assay blank. Furthermore, it may vary strikingly with the materials in the incubation medium: the presence or absence of serum can make a substantial difference, and one which it is highly important to control in any assay system.

(2) *Incomplete separation of the bound complex*:   In the presence of an excess of antibody it would be expected that 100% of the tracer ligand would be bound, but this optimum is rarely achieved and figures of 70% or less are frequently encountered. Possible explanations of this include:

(*i*) A proportion of the binder and hence the binder–ligand complex behaves similarly to free ligand; for example, with a second-antibody technique in a radioimmunoassay (see § 6.3.5.1) the precipitation may be incomplete;

(*ii*) Impurities may be present in the tracer ligand which do not react with the binder and thus emerge in the free fraction (e.g., free iodide);

(*iii*) The process of separation may lead to dissociation of the bound complex; for example, separation systems depending on absorption of free ligand by charcoal, leaving the bound fraction in solution, may be vitiated by the fact that the charcoal 'competes' with the binder and thus strips ligand from the bound complex (see § 6.3.3 and Fig. 6.4).

The reason for failure to achieve optimal separation of the bound complex is likely to vary in different systems. It is, therefore, essential when setting up a new assay that several separation procedures be examined.

6.2. *Practicality of separation procedures*

Of the available separation procedures, the best in terms of overall efficiency (low assay blank and completeness of separation of bound fraction) are probably solid-phase and second-antibody systems. However, both of these have disadvantages of practicality which are discussed under the headings of speed, simplicity, applicability and cost, though the four are to some extent interrelated. Speed is desirable because, for many purposes, a result reported to the clinician today is more valuable than the same result reported tomorrow. In practice, most separation procedures take considerably less time thant the incubation of the primary reaction and therefore add little to the duration of the assay as a whole.

Simplicity is an important factor, because on this may well depend the total number of samples which can be processed by a single operator. Thus, if the separation step requires detailed handling of each tube – for instance, application to a chromatographic column or to an electrophoretic strip – the total number of tubes which can be handled is limited and sample throughput correspondingly reduced. Furthermore, there is a direct relationship between the complexity of a technique and its reproducibility. Fortunately, most current separation procedures involve simple addition of one reagent, mixing, centrifugation and counting of the precipitate or supernatant; on the grounds of convenience the former is usually preferred because it does not involve a quantitative transfer from the assay tube. Of the common techniques, the only one to involve more than this is the use of particulate solid-phase immunosorbents which may require several wash steps if optimum results are to be achieved.

Applicability – in the sense of a single procedure being applied to a wide variety of different assays – is desirable but not essential. The best examples of techniques fulfilling this criterion are second-antibody and binder coupled to solid-phase: these are universal procedures which can be used for the separation of any binder–ligand system.

The costs of a radioimmunoassay reside chiefly in labour and less in reagents and capital equipment. Nevertheless, the costs of separation procedures vary widely and, all other things being equal, should be taken into account when setting up an assay. The cheapest systems are those involving the addition of a chemical precipitating agent (e.g., PEG); the most expensive are those systems which are either labour-intensive (chromatography, electrophoresis), or require considerable effort in the initial preparation of reagents (solid-phase systems, second antibody).

6.3. Methods for the separation of bound and free ligand

The methods are summarised in Table 6.1.

TABLE 6.1

Methods for the separation of bound and free ligand in a binding assay

Method	Reference
Electrophoresis (chromatoelectrophoresis, starch gel, cellulose acetate, polyacrylamide)	Berson et al., 1956; Hunter and Greenwood, 1964
Gel filtration (column or batch)	Haber et al., 1965
Adsorption (charcoal, magnetisable charcoal, silicates, hydroxyapatite, protein-A-containing Staphylococci)	Herbert et al., 1965; Rosselin et al., 1966; Jonsson and Kronvall, 1972; Trafford et al., 1974; Danes and Gardner, 1978
Fractional precipitation (ethanol, dioxan, polyethylene glycol, sodium sulphate, ammonium sulphate, trichloroacetic acid)	Heding, 1966; Thomas and Ferin, 1968; Desbuquois and Aurbach, 1971; Grodsky and Forsham, 1960; Chard et al., 1971; Mitchell and Byron, 1971
Partition (aqueous two-phase)	Mattiasson, 1980
Second antibody precipitation (soluble and solid-phase)	Utiger et al., 1962; Morgan and Lazarow, 1963; Hales and Randle, 1963; Den Hollander and Schuurs, 1977
Solid-phase antibody (particles, magnetic particles, tubes, gel entrapment, polymerised antibody)	Wide and Porath, 1966; Catt and Tregear, 1967; Updike et al., 1973; Donini and Donini, 1969; Nye et al., 1976; Halpern and Borden, 1979
Immunoradiometric assays	Miles and Hales, 1968; Woodhead et al., 1974

6.3.1. Electrophoresis

Paper chromatoelectrophoresis was the first method described for the separation of the reactants in a radioimmunoassay (insulin — Yalow and Berson, 1960). Other electrophoretic techniques, including starch gel, polyacrylamide gel, and cellulose acetate, have also been used, but all such techniques are cumbersome and little used in routine practice.

6.3.2. Gel filtration

As the binder—ligand complex must be larger than the ligand, separation of the two phases can be achieved by molecular sieve chromatography on materials such as Sephadex and Biogel. Two approaches have been employed:

(1) The gel matrix is used in the form of a column: this procedure is rather complex for routine manual application (Giese and Nielsen, 1971), but has been used as part of the semi-automated Centria system (see Ch. 13).

(2) The gel is incorporated in the incubation medium (Fig. 6.2); low M_r material (free ligand) can then distribute freely both inside and outside the gel, whereas higher M_r material (the bound complex) cannot enter the gel and thus is segregated in a small part of the system.

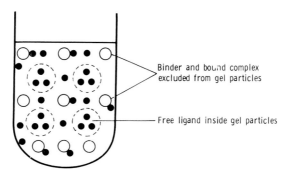

Fig. 6.2. Separation by the use of porous gel. Free ligand can enter the gel and will distribute between this and the liquid phase. Bound ligand is of higher M_r and is excluded from the gel.

Separation by batch addition of a gel or similar matrix was at one time widely used in commercial kits for the measurement of thyroid hormones.

6.3.3. Adsorption methods

The non-specific adsorption of biological molecules to particle surfaces is widely used as a method for the separation of bound and free ligand; most such procedures depend on the fact that only the ligand and not the binder or bound complex have this property (Fig. 6.3). In terms of the criteria for a separation technique, adsorption methods score highly on practicality (speed, simplicity and cost), but less highly on efficiency. Conditions (e.g., pH, temperature, ionic strength, protein concentration) must be carefully selected if adsorption of the bound complex is to be avoided; furthermore, if the binder–ligand complex has a high dissociation rate the adsorbent may compete for the ligand, thus effectively splitting the bound complex (Fig. 6.4).

The best known adsorption procedures are those using charcoal or silicates.

6.3.3.1. Charcoal   The use of powdered charcoal, for separation in a radioimmunoassay for insulin, was first described by Herbert et al. (1963), and has since been used in a wide variety of assays including competitive protein-binding assays. In its original form it was recom-

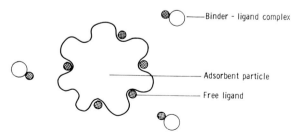

Fig. 6.3. Separation by the use of an adsorbent. Free ligand can enter 'crevices' on the particle and is firmly adsorbed. Bound ligand cannot enter the crevices and thus remains in the liquid phase.

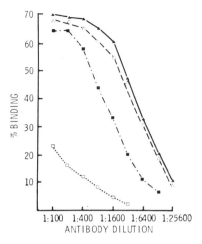

Fig. 6.4. The effect of different separation procedures on the apparent titre of an antiserum, in this case two different antisera to oxytocin, (tracer is ^{125}I-labelled oxytocin); separation is by the addition of ammonium sulphate (▲———▲, △———△), or charcoal (■—·—■, □·····□). The apparent titre is much lower with charcoal, since the latter can compete with the antibody for binding and thus 'strip' the bound complex.

mended that the charcoal be pre-treated with dextran of a given M_r-value. 'Coating' of this type was thought to block the larger pores which might accommodate the binder while not hindering the adsorption of the smaller M_r free ligand. It is likely that this concept is an over-simplification, since several workers have shown that the coating is unnecessary, particularly if serum is included in the incubation mixture (Ekins, 1969; Binoux and Odell, 1973).

The most commonly used of the available charcoals are the Norit range (Norit SXl) with a maximum particle size of 60 μm. Considerable batch-to-batch variation may be found with these, and it should never be assumed that the material in bottles with apparently identical labels will behave identically in an assay. Each batch should be carefully tested before it is put into routine use, and a high assay blank or low zero standard is an indication for testing another batch. A recent development with much promise is the use of 'magnetisable charcoal': charcoal and magnetisable ferric oxide trapped in a polyacrylamide gel, permitting separation by a magnet rather than centrifugation (Dawes and Gardner, 1978; Al-Dujaili et al., 1979). Some of the detailed procedures described in the literature demand close attention to factors such as molarity, temperature (operation at 4°C), and timing (centrifugation at a closely defined interval after addition of charcoal). For systems in which this degree of care is necessary, it is probably better to choose one of the many other separation procedures since exiguous requirements in the handling of the assay will inevitably, sooner or later, lead to errors and a loss of precision. A typical separation procedure using charcoal is shown in Table 6.2.

6.3.3.2. Silicates and hydroxyapatite

(1) *Particulate silicates*:   These have been used for separation in radioimmunoassay. Materials include talc, Quso G-32 (Calbiochem), Fuller's earth and Florisil. The principle of their operation is very similar to that of charcoal, as are their advantages and disadvantages. If they work well in a given system they are highly practical; if they do not, or demand close attention to detail, another procedure should be tried.

TABLE 6.2
A separation procedure using dextran-coated charcoal

(Radioimmunoassay of ACTH;   Rees et al., 1971)

1. Prepare a suspension containing 3.0 g of activated charcoal (Norit SXI — Hopkin and Williams Ltd.), 0.75 g Dextran T-70 (Pharmacia AB), 10 ml 0.5 M phosphate buffer (pH 7.4) 60 ml horse serum (Wellcome Reagents Ltd.), and 100 ml deionised water.
2. Stir the suspension on a magnetic stirrer.
3. After incubation of the primary reaction mixture (see Rees et al., 1971) add 0.2 ml of the charcoal suspension to each tube, mix, and centrifuge at 2000 x g for 15 min at 4°C or room temperature.
4. Aspirate the supernatant with a Pasteur pipette attached to a simple Venturi water pump.
5. Count the precipitate, containing the free fraction, by placing the tube in the well-crystal of a γ-counter.

(2) *Hydroxyapatite*:   With some systems, particularly steroid radioim-munoassays, hydroxyapatite (BDH Chemicals Ltd.) will adsorb the bound but not the free phase, thus providing a simple and rapid technique for separation (Trafford et al., 1974).

6.3.3.3. Protein-A-containing Staphylococci The surface of certain strains of *Staphylococcus* has a protein, 'protein-A', which is capable of binding the Fc part of an immunoglobulin molecule (see § 5.1.1). Preparations of these Staphylococci can rapidly (30 sec) bind immune complexes, and so permit removal of the bound fraction by centrifugation (Jonsson and Kronvell, 1972; Jonsson, 1978; Frohman et al., 1979). Protein-A has also been used as a 'universal tracer' in RIA systems (see § 3.8.1)

6.3.4. Fractional precipitation

Precipitation with salts or organic solvents was among the earliest methods for the fractionation of biological molecules. It is now widely applied for the separation of bound and free ligand in radioimmunoassays and related systems, and where it is appropriate, offers great practical advantages. The principal is simple. When the primary binder–ligand reaction is complete, the separation material is added to a concentration in which the binder and bound complex are insoluble and therefore precipitate, while the free fraction remains in solution. The precipitate is packed by centrifugation, and radioactivity determined either in the pellet (bound fraction) or the supernatant (free fraction).

The general mechanism of fractional precipitation depends on the use of salts and solvents which reduce the amount of 'free' water in a system: in other words, that water which is available to form a shell around a dissolved molecule and thus to keep it in solution (Fig. 6.5). For example, ammonium sulphate is capable of 'binding' water, which is then no longer available to form a shell for other molecules. Whether a substance will remain soluble at a given concentration of the separating agent is determined by its own ability to attract water molecules; for most biological materials the latter is determined by electrostatic charge and this, in turn by the isoelectric point and the pH of the medium. The greater the gap between these, the greater is the net charge which the molecule car-

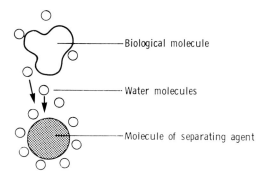

Fig. 6.5. The mechanism of action of precipitation of an antigen–antibody complex with ammonium sulphate. The latter takes up water molecules which are then not available to form a hydration shell for the protein.

ries and thus its ability to form water shells. Assay systems are conducted at or around neutral pH; increasing the concentration of salt or organic solvent will first precipitate those substances with an isoelectric point near neutrality, and then other materials in the order of their isoelectric points. The result is a fractionation very similar to that achieved by electrophoresis at the same pH, the slowest running molecules (with little net charge) being precipitated first. Molecules which are relatively hydrophobic (e.g., unconjugated steroid hormones, certain drugs) remain soluble even at very high concentrations of these separating agents.

Antibody molecules are γ-globulins which carry little charge at neutral pH and are therefore precipitated at low concentrations of reagents such as sodium sulphite (the first to be used in a radioimmunoassay system; Grodsky and Forsham, 1960), ammonium sulphate, ethanol, dioxane, and polyethylene glycol. Many antigens are not precipitated at these low concentrations, thus forming the basis for a simple and effective separation procedure.

Although the mechanism described above holds good for most systems there are, nevertheless, discrepancies, and whether or not a given reagent will produce an efficient separation is best determined experimentally. The type of experiment required is illustrated in Fig. 6.6. It is also found with some reagents (ammonium sulphate, polyethylene glycol) but not others (ethanol) that the antigen–antibody reaction will

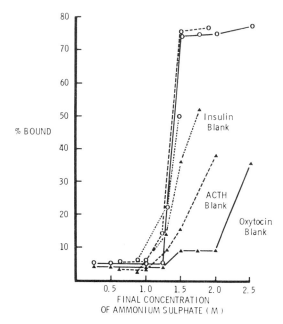

Fig. 6.6. An experiment to demonstrate the efficiency of a fractional precipitation procedure in assays for oxytocin, ACTH, and insulin. With oxytocin there is a substantial gap between the concentration of ammonium sulphate required to precipitate antibody-bound material and that which precipitates free antigen. With insulin, by contrast, there is almost no gap and this procedure would not be suitable for an assay.

continue in the presence of the reagent, i.e., with the antibody in precipitated form. Advantage can be taken of this in designing a system in which only a single addition of reagents is required — a mixture of tracer, binder and the separating agent.

In terms of efficiency the major problem of fractional precipitation methods is that they tend to yield a high assay blank, usually in the range of 5–20%. Not surprisingly, the extent of non-specific binding is somewhat related to the globulin concentration in the sample (Chen et al., 1980). The incorporation of a small amount of second antibody in the solution permits a lower concentration of the separating agent and

TABLE 6.3

Separation of bound and free ligand using polyethylene glycol

1. Prepare a 20% (w/v) solution of polyethylene glycol 6000 in phosphate buffer. Solution is speeded if a magnetic stirrer is used.
2. Add 2 volumes of this solution to the incubation mixture using a repeating syringe (i.e., 1 ml for the conditions shown in Tables 1.2 and 1.3).
3. Mix carefully on a vortex mixer to yield a homogeneous opalescent solution. There is no need to allow the suspension time to coagulate.
4. Centrifuge for 30 min at 2000 x *g* or greater. Temperature control is not necessary though results may be marginally improved at 4°C.
5. Decant or aspirate the supernatant. Aspiration, using a Pasteur pipette attached to a simple Venturi water pump, is usually preferable unless very wide base tubes are used.
6. Count the precipitate by placing the tube in the well crystal of a γ-counter.

Note: A very similar procedure would be followed using ethanol (2 volumes) or ammonium sulphate (1 volume of a saturated solution)

reduces the blank value without affecting the precipitation of the bound fraction.

In terms of practicality the fractional precipitation methods are superior to all others. They are simple, fast and cheap. For those assays to which they can be applied (almost all with the notable exception of those for very large protein molecules) they are highly reproducible, and batch-to-batch variation is virtually nil. A typical separation procedure using polyethylene glycol is shown in Table 6.3.

6.3.5. 'Double' antibody methods

6.3.5.1. 'Double' or 'second' antibody   Precipitation of the bound complex with an antibody directed to the binder is widely used as a separation procedure in radioimmunoassay systems, and was first introduced by Utiger et al. (1962) and Morgan and Lazarow (1963). The 'second' antibody is specific to the γ-globulin of the species in which the first antibody was raised — for example, if a guinea pig anti-insulin serum is used in the primary reaction of an assay for insulin, an antiserum to guinea pig γ-globulins raised in a goat might be used for the separation step (Fig. 6.7). Although most commonly used in radioimmunoassay, this concept could be applied to any binder.

Precipitation reactions occur only at high concentrations of antigen

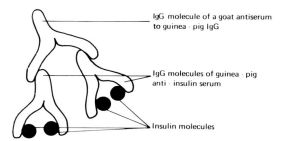

IgG molecule of a goat antiserum
to guinea - pig IgG

IgG molecules of guinea - pig
anti - insulin serum

Insulin molecules

Fig. 6.7. The principle of 'second-antibody' separation. With the addition of normal guinea pig serum to act as a carrier a precipitate is formed which includes the bound fraction.

and antibody; this is the reason why precipitation does not occur in most of the primary antigen—antibody reactions used in radioimmunoassay. Separation by this technique requires a relatively large concentration of second antibody and a correspondingly large amount of the species of γ-globulins of which the first antibody forms a part; for this purpose, a second antibody system always involves addition of carrier protein, either whole serum or γ-globulins from the species in which the first antibody was raised.

The initial design of a second-antibody separation technique follows principles similar to that of any immunological procedure used as a measurement system. A number of animals are immunised with γ-globulins, and their sera examined in experiments similar to that shown in Fig. 6.6 (i.e., precipitation of tracer in the presence and absence of antibody). In this case, however, it is necessary to test not only the concentration of antibody but also the appropriate concentration of carrier γ-globulins, since the optimal amounts will vary with each antiserum tested. Furthermore, with some antisera a significant proportion of the first antibody may be of the IgA or IgM classes and thus inadequately precipitated by a second antibody specific to IgG (Joyce et al., 1978). Selection of antiserum is critical, and the following factors should be investigated:

(1) Completeness of precipitation of the bound complex. In the presence of an excess of the first antibody this should represent as near as possible 100% of the immunoreactive tracer.

(2) The minimum quantity of 'second' antibody required to achieve complete precipitation. Excessive amounts are likely to be both expensive (see below) and to lead to the problem of the 'prozone' phenomenon — the fact that in the presence of an excess of antibody immunoprecipitation may not occur (Fig. 6.8).

(3) The 'assay blank' — the amount of tracer precipitated by second antibody in the absence of the first antibody. This should be less than 5%. A high value can occasionally be due to the presence in the antiserum of antibodies directed to the ligand.

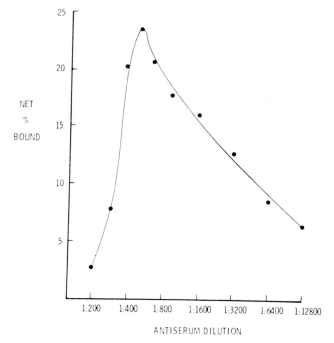

Fig. 6.8. The precipitation of ^{125}I-labelled LH (0.1 ng) by a rabbit anti-LH serum (final concentration 1:40,000) by a second antibody (goat anti-rabbit IgG). Normal rabbit serum (final concentration 1:20) was added as carrier. If the concentration of second antibody is too great (1:200) little or no precipitation occurs due to the prozone phenomenon. At 1:600 precipitation is optimal and at lower concentrations there is a progressive decline. In this system the concentration of second-antibody is therefore highly critical. (From data kindly supplied by Dr A.S. McNeilly.)

(4) The system should be evaluated in the presence of the fluid (e.g., plasma, serum, urine) for which the assay is designed. A procedure which appears satisfactory in the presence of diluent buffers may nevertheless, in the presence of biological materials, be subject to striking non-specific effects which are reflected as a reduction in precipitation of the bound complex or an increase in the assay blank or both. This is particularly likely to occur if the concentration of the sample exceeds 10% of the total volume in the assay tube. Interference in a second antibody system by plasma or serum has been attributed to the presence of high M_r globulins and complement (Morgan et al., 1964; Morgan, 1968). Materials used in the preparation of the sample (e.g., heparin, EDTA) may also be involved.

In terms of efficiency, a well-designed second antibody system is at least as good as and usually superior to most other separation procedures. It also has the advantage, in radioimmunoassays, of being a universal procedure. Thus, a satisfactory second antibody directed, for example, to rabbit globulins will be equally effective in all assays using a rabbit antiserum as the first antibody. However, the use of second antibody suffers from two important practical disadvantages:

(1) It requires an additional period of incubation which may range from 1–24 h, and can, therefore, considerably extend the time required to complete the assay. Incorporation of the second antibody with primary reagents, to yield a pre-precipitated complex (Hales and Randle, 1963; Wong et al., 1977; Brown et al., 1980), permits immediate separation and is increasingly applied. The rate of immunoprecipitation can be enhanced by incorporation of either ammonium sulphate or dextran with the second antibody (Martin and Landon, 1975); or 3–5% polyethylene glycol (Peterson and Swerdloff, 1979);

(2) Reagent supply: A new second antibody requires careful evaluation and may prove unsatisfactory. Relatively high concentrations are required, and the product of one animal is only sufficient for a limited number of assays. Second antibody systems are, therefore, expensive, regardless of whether the material is prepared locally or purchased from a commercial supplier (e.g., Wellcome Reagents Ltd.).

A typical separation procedure using second antibody is shown in Table 6.4.

TABLE 6.4

Separation of bound and free ligand using second antibody

The following recommendations are modified from the instruction leaflet of a commercial reagent (Wellcome Reagents Anti-Rabbit Globulin, code No. RD 17). This is chosen as an example because of its wide availability and excellent properties. It can be used with any system in which the antiserum to the ligand was raised in a rabbit.

1. Incorporate normal rabbit serum in the diluent buffer (0.1 ml/100 ml) to act as a carrier.
2. Following incubation of the primary reaction mixture add 0.1 ml of a dilution of the precipitating serum, and stand for a further 18 h at 4°C.
3. Centrifuge at 2000 x g or greater for 30 min.
4. Aspirate or decant the supernatant (Table 6.3).
5. Count the precipitate (Table 6.3).

Note: In the case of commercial reagents the appropriate dilution is usually stated with each batch. However, each user should check the exact conditions for his own assay (see text). In many cases it is possible to reduce the second incubation to as little as 2 h by adjustment of conditions.

6.3.5.2. Double-antibody solid-phase   Coupling of the second-antibody to an insoluble matrix such as cellulose (Den Hollander and Schuurs, 1971) yields a system which is convenient and which does not require the use of carrier γ-globulins. For the latter reason it is more economical of the second antibody itself. However, the preparation and evaluation is time-consuming, and the method is not widely used except in the form of commercially available reagent (Organon) or as part of an automated system (Centria, see § 13.5 and Meriadec et al., 1979).

6.3.6. Solid-phase systems

If the binder is covalently coupled to an insoluble support then both it and the bound complex can readily be separated from the soluble free fraction (Fig. 6.9). A wide variety of solid-phase supports have been described, which includes particles of dextran (Sephadex and Sepharose) and cellulose, and continuous surfaces such as polystyrene or polypropylene discs or the walls of plastic tubes. In terms of function, it is necessary to consider the two types separately.

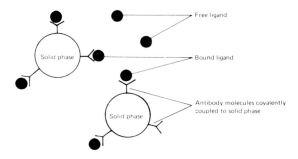

Fig. 6.9. Separation by the use of solid-phase coupled antibody.

6.3.6.1. Binder attached to discs, tubes and single glass beads   Plastic and glass surfaces exhibit absorptive properties, and exposing such surfaces to an appropriate dilution of an antiserum will lead to the attachment of a proportion of the antibody molecules (Catt and Tregear, 1967). Simple absorption is unlikely to involve covalent bonds and this may well explain the major drawback of earlier disc and tube systems — lack of reproducibility. This extends not only to the results in a single assay, but also to the initial choice of tube or disc which may vary considerably from batch to batch. A second drawback of coated tube systems is that the efficiency is rather less than that of other methods, since the total amount of tracer which can be bound by antibody excess is relatively low and the time required to reach equilibrium is extended. Although tube, disc and bead systems offer great convenience because centrifugation is not needed, they are only used in commercial kits in which the problems of reproducibility are avoided by the use of large and carefully screened batches of materials.

Considerable improvements can be made by linking the antibody covalently to the surface with glutaraldehyde (Appendix VI.4); the aldehyde groups form links between amino groups on the surface and those on the antibody. The number of amino groups on glass surfaces can be increased by pre-treatment with an amino-silane (Lynn, 1975) and a 'spacer' arm can be provided by pre-treating with aliphatic primary amines such as octadecylamine. Promising variations include the use of specially designed tube inserts, or single glass beads (Post et al., 1980).

6.3.6.2. Binder attached to particulate solid-phase   Particulate solid-phases are widely used. γ-Globulins from an antiserum are attached to the particles by a number of techniques which yield a covalent link between the protein and the particle, for example diazotisation or cyanogen bromide activation (Wide and Porath, 1966) (see Appendix VI.1). The resulting material is then extensively washed to ensure that no free γ-globulin molecules remain and is used as shown in Table 6.5. Interesting alternative approaches are the use of antibody entrapped in the interstices of a polyacrylamide gel (Updike et al., 1973), or nylon particles (Halpern and Bardens, 1979), or covalently bound to magnetic particles (polymer-coated iron oxide) (Nye et al., 1975). With the latter system mixing and separation can be simply achieved by the application of a magnetic field. Particulate solid-phases can also be used as supports for antigen (e.g., in an immunoradiometric assay, see § 6.4). With small molecules such as steroids or thyronines there may be steric interference due to the matrix, and in these cases a spacer molecule is placed between antigen and matrix. Materials with 6-carbon spacer arms are commercially available (e.g., AH-Sepharose 4B and CH-Sepharose 4B, Pharmacia,

TABLE 6.5
Use of solid-phase antibody for separation of bound and free ligand
(from Gardner et al., 1974)

1. Prepare antibody coupled to Sepharose as described in Appendix VI.1.
2. Prepare diluent buffer containing 0.1% (v/v) Tween 20 to prevent aggregation of the particles and non-specific adsorption of the tracer.
3. Set up the standard curve as shown in Table 1.3, but substituting a suspension of the solid phase for the soluble antibody. The appropriate dilution of the solid phase will vary between different antisera and must be established by experiment with different dilutions.
4. Cap all tubes and mix by vertical rotation (approx. 25 rev./min) for 1 h at room temperature.
5. Centrifuge at 2000 × g for 5 min, uncap the tubes, aspirate the supernatants leaving a constant volume (0.1 ml) in each tube, and wash once with 1 ml assay diluent.
6. Measure the counts in the solid phase by placing each tube in the well crystal of a γ-counter.
7. Calculate results (Table 1.2).

which use hexane as the 'spacer group'), and coupling is achieved by a one-step carbodiimide reaction (see Appendix VI.2).

A typical assay procedure using particulate solid-phase is shown in Table 6.5.

Solid-phase systems have several advantages:

(1) They can be applied to virtually any binder capable of covalent attachment to the particle;

(2) They are highly efficient and yield virtually complete separation of the bound fraction;

(3) They give excellent precision if carefully used;

(4) They are not as liable as some other systems to non-specific effects introduced by plasma and serum.

At the same time, solid-phase methods have certain disadvantages which explain why these sophisticated systems are not in universal use:

(1) The primary reagent is tedious to prepare;

(2) The recovery of antibody activity may be poor and is only acceptable if the supply of antiserum is abundant;

(3) In the case of antibodies to larger molecules, attachment to solid phase results in a loss of affinity and hence of sensitivity in the assay; this is only critical with that minority of assays in which extreme sensitivity is required;

(4) Most importantly, the actual assay procedure is more complex than with some other systems; for continuous mixing the tubes must be capped and uncapped; at the end of the procedure the washing of the solid phase sometimes involves several steps of centrifugation and aspiration.

Thus, for any assay with a large sample throughput, particulate solid-phase systems are not technically convenient.

6.3.7. Conclusions – the choice of a separation procedure

There is no magic in any one separation procedure. For a given assay system the choice potentially embraces all the techniques described above, and there is no reason to follow slavishly an earlier published technique. Instances abound of the perpetuation of a complex and sometimes inefficient method simply because it was the first to be described. For example, charcoal separation continues to be used in assays for steroids and small peptides, systems in which dissociation of the bound complex is very likely to occur and thus impair efficiency. Other systems offering equal and probably greater convenience are available and should be used.

There is much to be said for keeping the number of separation systems in any one laboratory to a minimum. Two or three general techniques whose characteristics are well-understood and for which the reagents are freely available are clearly preferable to a multitude of different methods each with their own particular faults. In terms of radioimmunoassay the two techniques which have best stood the test of time are chemical precipitation and the use of second antibody. Faced with setting up a new radioimmunoassay, and assuming that the primary reagents are known to be appropriate, the worker would be well advised to explore the use of a simple precipitation system — for example, polyethylene glycol (Table 6.3). If it is not possible to optimise a method of this type, for the reasons set out above, then a second-antibody system should be examined (Table 6.4), possibly with the addition of polyethylene glycol to enhance the rate. In this author's experience there is no assay for which one or the other systems has not proved highly satisfactory.

It should never be assumed that any separation technique is perfect and produces total separation of the free and bound fraction; nor should it be assumed that, in terms of function, separation techniques differ only in their efficiency. The observation that two different procedures yield identical results for assay blank and zero standard does not necessarily mean that the composition of these fractions is identical: for example, much of the assay blank might consist in the one case of damaged tracer, and in the other of intact tracer precipitated because of an overlap between the characteristics of the bound and free fractions. Such a difference could yield a striking discrepancy between the actual assay results yielded by the two methods (see § 10.2.4). Finally, it should be emphasised that the results obtained with any separation procedure are almost certain to vary with the actual medium used in the assay (e.g., serum, plasma, urine). Comparison of standards, prepared in a diluent buffer, with unknowns, which are serum samples, will usually reveal non-identity which is in reality an artefact of the separation technique. The only solution to this problem is to ensure that standards are prepared in media as near as possible identical to that of the sample: for instance, in hormone-free serum where this is available (see § 10.3.4).

6.4. Immunoradiometric techniques (IRMA)

The elegant technique of immunoradiometric assay (Miles and Hales, 1968; Woodhead et al., 1974) is considered in this chapter because it represents an important variant in which bound and free binder are separated rather than bound and free ligand. Reflection on the basic equations for binding assay systems (see § 1.4) will reveal that there is no truly fundamental difference between the two approaches, since the distinctions between binder and ligand are operational rather than real; it does not affect the basic logic of the system if the terms binder and ligand are reversed. However, it has been argued that IRMA systems *are* fundamentally different because they sometimes involve the use of an excess of labelled reagent, whereas conventional systems always use limiting reagent (see Ekins, 1980 and § 9.2.12). But whatever the theoretical arguments, the technique does have major potential advantages.

The technique of a classical radiometric assay is summarised in Fig. 6.10. A preliminary step is to isolate and label specific antibodies to the ligand. An antiserum is extracted with an immunoadsorbent made by coupling highly purified antigen to a solid phase such as cellulose or Sepharose (see Appendix VI for details of coupling reactions). The antiserum is mixed with the solid-phase antigen and after equilibration the serum is removed, leaving only specific antibodies attached to the solid-phase antigen. As with other solid-phase systems (see above) extensive washing is essential at every step to ensure that no soluble material remains. The antibodies are then iodinated in situ on the solid phase using a standard chloramine-T procedure and sufficient ^{125}I to yield a substitution rate of 1—2 iodine atoms/antibody molecule. Residual iodide and damaged products are removed by further washing of the solid phase followed by elution from the immunoadsorbent of low-affinity antibodies at pH 3 and higher-affinity antibodies at pH 2. The purified labelled antibodies are collected into a neutral buffer and then stored until use either in this form, or after recombination with the immunoadsorbent to improve their stability. An alternative approach is to pre-

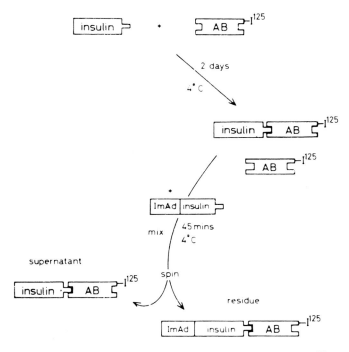

Fig. 6.10. The immunoradiometric assay of Miles and Hales (1968). ^{125}I-labelled, purified antibody to insulin is incubated with sample or standard. Free antibody is then separated by the addition of insulin coupled to a solid phase (ImAd). The greater the amount of insulin in sample or standard, the smaller will be the amount of antibody bound in the solid phase (Fig. 6.11).

pare immunoglobulins from the antiserum and to iodinate these *prior* to immunosorption; however, this is very wasteful of ^{125}I since only some 2–3% will be recovered with the purified antibodies.

In the IRMA assay itself (Fig. 6.10) samples and standards are incubated with an appropriate concentration of the purified antibody (determined by experiment). After equilibration unreacted antibody is removed by addition of an excess of the immunoadsorbent which after further incubation is removed, washed, and counted. The greater the amount of ligand in the assay tube, the greater will be the amount of

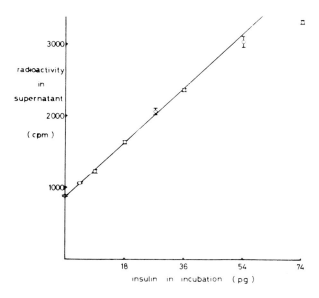

Fig. 6.11. A standard curve for an immunoradiometric assay, performed according to the principle shown in Fig. 6.10.

tracer antibody which forms a soluble complex and is therefore not available to bind to the immunoadsorbent. The result is a standard curve (Fig. 6.11) in which the number of counts in the supernatant is directly proportional to the amount of ligand present.

Apart from technical complexity, the 'classical' immunoradiometric assay has one important drawback: non-reactive material in the labelled antibody preparation (i.e., damaged components) will be present in the zero standard and can thus lead to a high baseline response. This may explain why the original procedure has found little practical application, and why the future almost certainly lies with the 'two-site' techniques described below.

The major variation on the immunometric procedure is the so-called 'two-site' or 'sandwich' assay (Addison and Hales, 1971) which employs unlabelled antibody coupled to a solid phase together with the liquid phase purified antibodies already described. Procedures of this type have been described for several antigens and are the basis of a commercial kit for the assay of TSH (Immunophase, Corning). They may avoid some of the non-specific effects arising from factors in the biological fluid; they permit an increase in sensitivity since relatively large volumes of the fluid can be extracted; and because the solid phase is counted this can be washed free of non-reactive components to yield a very low baseline noise signal.

A number of protocols have been examined with two-site assays (Table 6.6). In addition, the use of labelled second antibodies has been described (Hales et al., 1975; Fruchard et al., 1978), another example of a universal tracer (see § 3.8.1). Systems of this type could be of great value where the supply of first antibody is limited.

6.4.1. Advantages of the immunoradiometric assay

The advantages of the immunoradiometric assay are as follows:
(1) Iodination of the antigen is avoided, and with it the problems of damage to the tracer arising either during preparation or incubation (see § 3.7.4); antibodies are large and relatively stable molecules and therefore less liable to damage;

TABLE 6.6
Variations on immunometric assays

Immunoradiometric assay	Liquid-phase purified ^{125}I-labelled antibody and solid-phase antigen
'Two-site' immunoradiometric assay	Liquid phase purified ^{125}I-labelled antibody and solid-phase antibody
— antigen reacted with solid-phase antibody followed by reaction with ^{125}I-labelled antibody	
— simultaneous reaction of antigen with solid-phase antibody and ^{125}I-labelled antibody	
— antigen reacted with ^{125}I-labelled antibody, followed by reaction with solid-phase antibody	

(2) If the antibody is iodinated as a complex with the immunoadsorbent, the combining site is protected;

(3) The procedure can be applied to materials which are difficult to iodinate – for example, peptides lacking a tyrosine residue;

(4) The procedure is of great value for assays in which highly purified antigen for labelling is in short supply, while specific antibody is abundant. An example is TSH: a very small amount of pure material suffices for immunisation and the production of large quantities of specific antibody; purified antibody can then be prepared on an immunosorbent of relatively crude TSH. These procedures are ideal for the use of monoclonal antibodies (see § 5.3) since the latter require little or no purification;

(5) Immunometric assays lend themselves very well to the use of non-isotopic labels (Ch. 4);

(6) Because it is possible to select high-affinity antibodies from a heterogeneous population in the antiserum, the procedure may be more sensitive than conventional techniques;

(7) Provided that the dissociation constant of the primary reaction is low, the procedure lends itself to 'tracer excess' systems and thus to very rapid assays, or to much enhanced sensitivity, *unrelated* to the affinity of the antibody (see § 9.2.12);

(8) In the 'two-site' assay it is possible to select and estimate only those molecules which contain both antigenic sites.

The advantages of immunoradiometric assay over conventional RIA have been clearly demonstrated in an assay for alphafetoprotein (Hunter and Budd, 1981): the working range for the IRMA was 4-fold wider and the detection limit 10-fold lower.

The disadvantages of immunoradiometric assays are:

(1) Preparation of the basic materials can be time-consuming and require a high level of technical expertise;

(2) As with other solid-phase systems, the consumption of reagent is high because of the losses associated with coupling and purification; for this reason, the technique is not suitable for assays in which the supply of basic material is limited;

(3) Most present 'two-site' systems are in reality 'pseudo two-site' because the same antibody is used in both the solid and liquid phases. A true 'two-site' system would employ antibodies to *separate* antigenic determinants on the ligand.

Because of their practical disadvantages immunoradiometric systems are still not widely applied. The most notable exception is the two-site system for hepatitis B antigen ('AUSRIA', Abbott Laboratories) which has the great advantage that it avoids the use of a potentially infectious standard antigen. However, further applications of the 'two-site' assays are likely in the future, more particularly since the production of 'monoclonal' antibodies has now become a practical proposition; an example of such an assay has been described for α-fetoprotein (Uotila et al., 1981).

CHAPTER 7

Requirements for binding assays – extraction of ligand from biological fluids and collection and storage of samples

In most radioimmunoassays the procedure consists of simple addition and mixing of sample, tracer, and binder. However, there are situations in which this does not suffice, and the sample must be processed prior to its introduction into the assay:

– If the assay does not have sufficient sensitivity and endogenous ligand must therefore be concentrated;

– If the assay does not have sufficient specificity and endogenous ligand must therefore be separated from other materials.

These demands can be met by a variety of extraction procedures (Table 7.1).

TABLE 7.1

Extraction procedures used in association with binding assays

Procedure	Main purpose
Extraction with particulate adsorbents	Increasing the sensitivity of assays of small peptides
Extraction with immunosorbents	Increasing the sensitivity and specificity of any assay; 'two-site' immunometric assays
Extraction with organic solvents	Increasing the specificity of assays for haptens such as steroid hormones (can also increase sensitivity)
Extraction with cellulose filters	Detection of airborne industrial contaminants (e.g., papain; Wells et al., 1981)
Dissociation procedures	Conversion of steroid conjugates to native form; elimination of endogenous binding proteins
Treatment with detergents	Exposure of antigenic sites on lipoproteins (Maciejko and Mao, 1982)

7.1. General aspects of extraction procedures

Virtually the whole range of physicochemical procedures used in the purification of biological materials might be applicable as extraction procedures for an assay. However, the practical criteria for use with a routine assay may include the following:

(1) Speed and simplicity, to match the large number of determinations which may be required;

(2) Concentration of the ligand into a volume considerably smaller than that of the original sample, to improve sensitivity;

(3) Elimination of non-specific interfering factors to improve specificity;

(4) Reproducible recovery of 50% or more of the original ligand;

(5) No significant alteration of the ligand;

(6) The materials used should be readily available and should not vary from batch to batch.

It cannot be emphasised too strongly that extraction procedures may yield results which vary considerably both in different laboratories, and (from time to time) in the same laboratory. Even if a system has been clearly described in the literature it must be carefully re-checked according to the following criteria:

(1) *Recovery*:   This is presented as the percentage of a fixed amount of ligand recovered. The optimum is 100%, but figures greater than 50% are acceptable; a simple and reproducible technique with a recovery of 60% is preferable to a complex and variable procedure with a recovery of 90%. Recovery should always be studied for different concentrations of the ligand, chosen to cover the range which is likely to be encountered in biological fluids. Experimental evaluation of recovery is simplified by the use of labelled ligand, though it should not be assumed that this behaves identically with unlabelled ligand.

(2) *Reproducibility*:   This should be reported as the coefficient of variation of repeated determinations on the same sample. At least 10 observations are required for the figure given to have any validity, and it should be based on the results of experiments performed on separate occasions by different operators. It is particularly important to note whether the recovery varies significantly from one run to the next;

'significantly' in this context means as a result of the performance of a '*t*' or '*F*' test, not simply glancing through the data. If the difference between occasions is not significant then there is no need to run recovery controls with every assay – representing a considerable saving of time and materials. If the difference is significant then a separate recovery experiment is always necessary, as is commonly practised with steroid hormone assays.

(3) *Identity of extracted and unextracted ligand*:   The manipulations involved in the extraction process can introduce two types of non-identity. Either the ligand itself is physicochemically altered, so that it no longer reacts in the same way with the binder; or the extract contains materials which interfere with the binder–ligand reaction. The most obvious result of non-identity is non-parallelism between dilutions of the unextracted ligand (standard) and the extracted ligand. This might reflect damage to some but not all of the different binding sites on the ligand. Alternatively, it might be due to a completely non-specific chemical effect on the reaction such as that illustrated in Fig. 7.1. But it is very important to recognise that parallelism does not guarantee identity (see § 10.2.2). Thus, partial damage to a single binding site, with a reduction

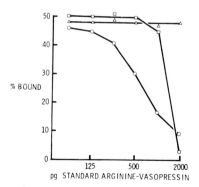

Fig. 7.1. Non-specific non-specificity resulting from an extraction procedure (absorption and elution of arginine-vasporessin from glass beads, Table 7.2): (o———o), standard curve; (△———△), serial dilutions of a plasma extract; (□———□), serial dilutions of the same plasma extract which had not been adequately neutralised by washing (i.e., the antigen–antibody reaction was inhibited by acid pH).

in affinity between binder and ligand, will decrease the apparent potency of the extracted ligand but will not lead to non-parallelism. Similarly, there is no a priori reason to suppose that interference due to completely non-specific factors will always lead to non-parallelism of the type shown in Fig. 7.1. Given apparent parallelism between extract and standard, final proof of identity can only be obtained from an experiment in which each of the standards is also separately extracted. For the reasons given below, the experiment has to be conducted using standard added to biological fluid (e.g., plasma or urine) which is known to be free of endogenous ligand.

(4) *Blank value*:   It is often found that extracts of a biological fluid, known to be free of the ligand, will nevertheless give a positive value when read against a standard curve prepared in a simple aqueous buffer solution. In some instances it is possible to recognise easily this 'blank' value as an artefact − for example, if the ligand under investigation is a drug, then samples from untreated subjects should definitely give a zero reading. In other instances, identification is less simple − for example, with basal levels of an endogenous hormone. 'Hormone free' samples can be obtained by two means: either from patients known to lack the hormone because the organ of origin has been destroyed; or by appropriate treatment of the sample with adsorbents known to remove the hormone. Neither type of sample is completely satisfactory. To guarantee that a patient has none of a certain hormone is rarely absolute; for example, many subjects who have had what should be a complete ablation of the pituitary will nevertheless continue to have normal or elevated circulating levels of prolactin. Artificial preparation of the sample by absorption of the hormone (as with charcoal for the production of insulin-free plasma) may be highly efficient but could easily have secondary effects on other components of the fluid which would eliminate a non-specific blank at the same time. It can never therefore be certain whether the blank is a true basal level, or an artefact. Other studies, including changes under well-defined physiological circumstances, and a formal physicochemical identification of the extracted material, should thus be performed.

7.2. *Extraction using particulate adsorbents*

Extraction with particulate adsorbents is widely used for the concentration of small peptide hormones (e.g., ACTH and vasopressin) whose concentrations in body fluids are at or below the minimum detection limits of a fully optimised radioimmunoassay. The principle of concentration by extraction is illustrated in Fig. 7.2: the procedure can be applied to a relatively large volume of fluid and yields a final volume of extract which is very much smaller. Specificity may also be improved since the procedure can separate the ligand from interfering materials including proteolytic enzymes (see § 10.3).

The commonly used adsorbents are all particulate silicates (e.g., Fuller's earth, glass beads, silicic acid). These materials have in common a large surface area in relation to their weight. The precise nature of the adsorption process is uncertain. Rather more specific, in that the nature of the adsorption process is understood, is the use of concanavalin A linked to agarose for extraction of glycoproteins — for example, TSH

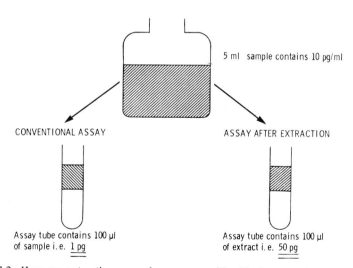

Fig. 7.2. How an extraction procedure can considerably increase the sensitivity of a binding assay.

from serum (Nisula et al., 1978). An example of extraction using a particulate adsorbent is shown in Table 7.2.

The 'two-site' immunoradiometric assay (see § 6.4) is also an example of the use of an adsorbent for extraction, though in this case the process is completely specific because it depends on a solid-phase antibody rather than non-specific adsorption to a surface. Solid-phase antibody has also been used as an adsorbent in a conventional radioimmunoassay for vaso-pressin (Morton and Riegger, 1978) and ethinyloestradiol (Dyas et al., 1981), for a fluroimmunoassay of thyroxine (Nargessi et al., 1980) and for prostatic acid phosphatase prior to conventional enzyme determination (Lee et al., 1980). Further applications of this attractive approach may be expected in the near future.

7.3. Extraction with organic solvents

There are many instances in the field of binding assays in which ambi-guity may arise because of the presence of closely related materials in biological fluids and sometimes it is not possible to overcome this by the

TABLE 7.2

An extraction and concentration procedure using a particulate adsorbent

(Radioimmunoassay of ACTH, modified from Rees et al., 1971)

1. To 2.5 ml plasma in a plastic tube add 50 mg Vycor glass (Corning Glass Works).
2. Cap tubes and mix by rotation for 30 min.
3. Centrifuge ($2000 \times g$ for 5 min); aspirate and discard the supernatant.
4. Wash the precipitate with 3 ml deionised water, then 2 ml of 1 M HCl.
5. Mix solid with 2 ml 60% (v/v) acetone in deionised water to elute ACTH.
6. Centrifuge, carefully remove supernatant with a Pasteur pipette and transfer to a plastic tube.
   N.B. A different pipette should be used for each sample.
7. Place the tube in a sandbath or waterbath at 50°C and evaporate to dryness with a fine jet of oxygen-free nitrogen.
8. Dissolve the residue in 0.5 ml diluent buffer for radioimmunoassay.

Note: The procedure described is specific to the ACTH assay but with small varia-tions can be used for a variety of small peptide hormones use of highly specific binders. In the case of small hapten molecules, such as the steroid hormones, preliminary extraction of the ligand from an aqueous biological fluid into an organic solvent can much improve the specificity of the assay. This is particularly the case in assays which use naturally occurring binding proteins as the binder; these proteins are likely to show a broad range of specificity (see § 5.5) and two examples will serve to show the use of extraction to overcome the problem.

(1) *Measurement of progesterone using transcortin as the binding agent*: Transcortin will bind a variety of corticosteroids and other steroids in addition to progesterone. In order to achieve specificity, prior extraction of the sample with solvents such as petroleum—ether, which selectively takes up progesterone, permits unambiguous determination of this steroid (Johansson, 1969).

(2) *Measurement of androgens using sex-hormone binding globulin as binding agent*: SHBG will bind a variety of 17 β-hydroxy-C-19 steroids, including both testosterone and oestradiol. A simple solvent extraction permits the separation and determination of 'testosterone-like' substances (Anderson, 1970) which, though still a mixture, nevertheless provides a practical reflection of androgenic activity.

Some type of solvent extraction is considered to be essential for all steroid hormones, with the possible exception of those which circulate at very high levels. This applies equally to radioimmunoassays of high specificity and competitive protein binding assays of low specificity. Attempts to eliminate the extraction step, while highly commendable from the point of view of practicality, can often lead to over-estimates of low levels and to non-specific effects due to materials such as fatty acids (Greiner et al., 1978). An example of a solvent extraction for a steroid assay is shown in Table 7.3.

Certain general points can be made about solvent extraction:

(1) Solvents must be of the highest possible purity and checked frequently by, for example, evaporating solvent alone and determining the 'blank' value in the assay. Any new method must be rigorously evaluated according to the criteria already set out above.

TABLE 7.3

An extraction procedure using organic solvents

(Radioimmunoassay of progesterone, method kindly supplied by Dr K.K. Dighe)

1. To 1 ml serum in a glass tube (approx. 16 x 75 mm) add 3 pg [³H]progesterone (approx. 2000 dpm) (Radiochemical Centre); mix and stand for 2 h or overnight at 4°C.
2. Add 0.1 ml ethanol; mix and leave for 15 min at 4°C.
3. Add 10 ml petroleum ether (AR grade; 40–60°C boiling point) and shake for 10 min (multiple tube shakers are available for this purpose; e.g., Baird and Tatlock).
4. Allow the organic (upper) and aqueous layers to separate.
5. Freeze the aqueous layer by placing the tube in a mixture of dry ice/acetone.
6. Transfer the organic layer to a separate tube and place in a water-bath at 50–60°C for 5–6 h until dry.
7. Redissolve the extract in 1 ml assay buffer and leave for 2 h at 4°C to ensure complete solution.
8. Remove 0.5 ml; add 4 ml liquid scintillation mixture and count in a liquid scintillation counter* to ascertain percentage recovery [(added counts/2) x (recovered counts/100)].
9. Remove duplicate 0.1 ml aliquots for progesterone RIA**.

* A liquid scintillation mixture can be prepared by dissolving 4 g of 2,5-diphenyloxazole (PPO) in 600 ml toluene (analytical grade) and 400 ml Triton X-100 (scintillation grade). Appropriate mixtures are also available commercially (e.g., Aquafluor, Riafluor; New England Nuclear). For details of liquid scintillation counting see vol. 5 of this series (Fox, 1976)
** A typical protocol would be 0.1 ml extract + 0.1 ml [³H]progesterone (approx. 30 pg, 20,000 dpm) + 0.1 ml antibody to progesterone (ILS Ltd.); leave for 2 h at 4°C; separate bound and free with dextran-coated charcoal (see Table 6.2); transfer an aliquot of the supernatant (bound fraction) for liquid scintillation counting

(2) The solvent should be optimised for each individual steroid according to its polarity. For example, extraction of progesterone with hexane may yield cleaner material than does extraction with a more polar solvent such as ether (see Jeffcoate, 1978).

(3) Current developments are improving the convenience of solvent extraction. For example, separation of the aqueous and organic phases is made much simpler by freezing the aqueous phase in a mixture of

solid CO_2 and acetone, following which the organic supernatant can be decanted (Table 7.3). Purpose-built equipment is now available for evaporation of large numbers of tubes in a steam of air or nitrogen.

In some cases solvent extraction alone does not yield adequate specificity, and chromatographic separation has to be included. Chromatography also has an important place in the initial validation of an assay and can be used for the determination of multiple individual steroids in a single sample. Earlier methods based on paper or thin-layer chromatography are unsatisfactory because of the instability of picogram amounts of steroids during the drying process. They have been replaced by the use of column chromatography on hydrophobic matrices such as Sephadex LH-20 (Pharmacia) (Murphy, 1971; Sippel et al., 1978) or Lipidex 5000 (hydroxyalkoxypropyl-Sephadex, Pharmacia) (Hammond et al., 1977), or high-performance liquid chromatography (Schoneshofer et al., 1981). These techniques have the advantage of speed, high recoveries, excellent

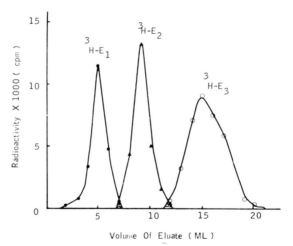

Fig. 7.3. Separation of tritiated oestrone (●——●), oestradiol (△——△), and oestriol (○——○) (all in 0.1 ml containing 50,000 cpm) on a 10 cm x 0.5 cm column of Sephadex LH-20 eluted with chloroform:hexane:methanol (46:46:8, by vol.). This type of separation, applied to a plasma extract, permits specific quantitation of any of the three oestrogens using a relatively non-specific binding assay (data kindly supplied by Dr S. Khoshroo).

reproducibility, low blank values, and convenience because the same column can be used several times. An example of the sort of separation which can be achieved is shown in Fig. 7.3.

7.4. Dissociation procedures

Endogenous ligand in a biological fluid may be in a form not directly accessible to the assay — for example, as a conjugate, or as a complex with a circulating binding protein.

7.4.1. Conversion of conjugated steroids to the unconjugated forms

With most steroid hormones a significant fraction circulates as sulphate or glucuronide conjugates, and these will not react in assays directed towards the unconjugated material. In the case of oestriol in late pregnancy plasma 90% or more of the steroid may be in this form. Hydrolysis of steroid conjugates in preparation for binding assays follows exactly the same principles as those applied to the classical fluorimetric or gas chromatographic procedure. The sample is treated with either strong acid* or a hydrolytic enzyme**, and the steroid thus freed is extracted for assay. The advantage of enzyme hydrolysis is that, if the levels of the hormone are sufficiently high, the final extraction step may be unnecessary. An alternative to hydrolysis is the use of radioimmunoassays which are specific to the conjugate as a whole (e.g., to oestriol-16-glucuronide). This approach is theoretically very attractive since it eliminates a time-consuming step which is also a potential source of error (Collins and Hennan, 1976).

---

* Preedy and Aitken (1961), 5–15 ml plasma, diluted to 100 ml with water plus 17.5 ml conc. HCl, is refluxed for 45 min

** *Helix pomatia* extract (containing glucuronidase and sulphatase (available from Calbiochem)

7.4.2. Dissociation of ligand from endogenous binding proteins

Complexing with circulating binding proteins is well-illustrated by the steroids, and also with the hormones of the thyroid gland. The endogenous binder, which is usually at high concentrations, will compete with assay binder for both ligand and tracer ligand. As a result, a large part of the endogenous ligand is inacessible to the assay, and also the endogenous binding will compete for the tracer and limit the sensitivity of the assay (Fig. 7.4). Depending on the nature of the assay binder (i.e., naturally occurring binding protein or antibody) and on the separation procedure used, the eventual result will be either a very low apparent level or a very high level, both equally unrelated to the circulating level of the hormone. A wide variety of methods have been described for freeing ligand from binding proteins: examples are shown in Table 7.4.

Another situation in which an endogenous binder can affect assay results is in the study of samples containing actively-produced antibodies to the ligand. This may occur as a result of a planned immunisation in animals or as an unintended side-effect of therapy in the human. For example, most patients on long-term therapy with hormones from natural sources (growth hormone, insulin, posterior pituitary extracts) will develop antibodies to these materials. In terms of the assay of endogenous ligand this has two effects:

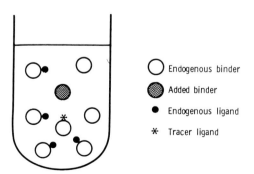

Endogenous binder
Added binder
Endogenous ligand
Tracer ligand

Fig. 7.4. The need for a dissociation procedure when the sample contains an endogenous binder. The latter will compete with the assay binder for both endogenous and tracer ligand, thus invalidating any results obtained.

TABLE 7.4

Examples of procedures for freeing ligand from endogenous binding proteins

Ligand	Procedure	Reference
Steroid hormones	Solvent extraction of sample	See § 7.3
Steroid hormones	Displacement with unrelated steroids	Jurjens et al., 1975
Steroid hormones	Operation of assay at low pH (3.5)*	Rolleri et al., 1976
Steroid hormones	Enzyme digestion of proteins	Hasler et al., 1975
Thyroxine	Extraction of sample with ethanol	Murphy, 1965
Thyroxine	Incorporation of anilino-napthalene sulphonic acid (ANS) (1 mg/ml) in assay*	Chopra, 1972
Thyroxine	Operation of assay at low pH (4.0)*	Gartner et al., 1980
Vitamin B12	Heating the sample (100°C) at acid pH	Leonard and Beckers, 1975
Vitamin B12	Pre-treatment of sample with alkali (pH 13.6)	Ithakissios et al., 1980

* This inhibits the endogenous–ligand reaction, but not the antibody–ligand reaction

(1) Binding of the tracer by high levels of antibody in the sample will yield either very low or zero results;

(2) The presence of a circulating antibody, which will often negate the biological effect of the hormone, may be associated with total hormone levels which are in reality exceptionally high.

The measurement of total hormone under these circumstances demands a preliminary extraction step. In practice, and depending on the nature of the material studied, this might involve any of the types of procedure already discussed. A more general method, which can in principle be applied to any material, is to dissociate the endogenous antigen—antibody complex with acid, and then to submit the sample to gel chromatography which will separate the free antibody and the free antigen.

7.4.3. Other uses of dissociating agents

Problems with the specificity of the primary reagents are not confined to the steroid hormones. Other instances arise with the proteins and peptides, particularly where these exist in different molecular forms in biological fluids. For example, low levels of carcino-embryonic antigen (CEA) can only be examined after prior removal of interfering materials by perchloric acid precipitation or heating (Nishi and Hirai, 1975).

7.5. Measurement of 'free' hormones

A specialised example of separation of ligand from endogenous binding protein is the measurement of 'free' hormones. In this situation the aim is to measure only that fraction which is not protein bound in the circulation, i.e., the fraction which is usually considered to be responsible for biological activity. Such a measurement can, in principle, eliminate the ambiguities which may arise from the estimation of total concentration because of variations in the amount of binding protein present. For example, subjects receiving oestrogen-containing oral contraceptive agents have elevated levels of thyroxine-binding globulin (TBG); total thyroxine levels are correspondingly increased, but the free fraction remains unaltered. The measurement of 'free' biologically active levels of a hormone can be achieved by subjecting the serum sample to equilibrium

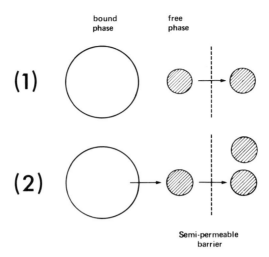

Fig. 7.5. Why it may be impossible to obtain a true level of a 'free' hormone. All separation methods involve a semi-permeable barrier which allows passage of free hormone but not bound (this is equally true of dialysis, ultrafiltration, gel-filtration, and distribution into porous particles). When the free phase has diffused across this barrier (1), the Law of Mass Action dictates that some bound hormone will dissociate and enter the free pool (2). Eventually a new equilibrium will be reached when the concentration of free hormone is the same on both sides of the barrier. At this point, the total free hormone will be considerably greater than it was in the original sample.

dialysis (Sterling and Hegedus, 1962), ultrafiltration (Thorson et al., 1972), or gel filtration (Irvine, 1972) to separate free from bound hormone. The distribution is assessed by the inclusion of a small amount of tracer hormone in the system, or by direct assay of the hormone in the free phase. All systems suffer from the disadvantage that some of the bound hormone may dissociate during the separation procedure, thus leading to overestimates of the free form (Fig. 7.5); this explains the very wide range of estimates which have been made of the absolute levels of free hormones, and may also explain why the clinical value of these estimates is often little superior to that of total hormone. An interesting new approach to measurement of 'free' hormone is observation of the kinetics of desorption of tracer from endogenous binder to a solid-phase antibody (Hertl and Odstrchel, 1978). This technique has a better theoretical basis than existing methods, and is considerably more rapid and practical. Another approach, which is at the biological rather than the technical level, is to examine hormone levels in saliva (Walker et al., 1978). The hormone content in this site represents a 'transudate' of the free hormone levels in the circulation.

7.6. Conclusions – the elimination of extraction procedures

Though widely used in many common assays, extraction procedures must be regarded as inherently undesirable:

(1) They inevitably lead to a loss of precision due to the summation of errors with every additional step;

(2) Most importantly, they drastically limit the number of samples which can be processed by a single operator. The addition of 2 or 3 reagents to a measured volume of sample in a straightforward non-extraction radioimmunoassay takes 20 sec or less, whereas none of the procedures described in this chapter takes less than 3–4 min of direct operator time. Throughputs of 100 or more samples per day may be reduced to a dozen.

For all these reasons, extraction procedures should be regarded as an expedient, to be replaced whenever possible by a non-extraction technique. Possible approaches include:

(1) The production of better antibodies (with respect to affinity or specificity or both);

(2) Changes in assay protocol – such as the incorporation of dissociating agents in the assay buffer (§ 7.4.2.);

(3) Consideration of whether the problem which dictates the need for an extraction procedure is in fact a real problem – for example, in the measurement of blood oestriol in late pregnancy it is actually immaterial whether the assay measures conjugated or unconjugated hormone, or even a mixture of the two; convenience and reproducibility are far more important than absolute specificity.

7.7. *Sample collection for radioimmunoassay*

This is an appropriate point at which to consider some general aspects of sample collection for radioimmunoassay. The primary aim is to ensure that the material which goes into the assay tube is as near as possible identical to that which was present in the circulation of the patient. Sometimes (but fortunately rarely) an extraction procedure is necessary to achieve this. Far more frequently the assay is performed directly on serum or plasma (or other fluids) and the main potential difficulty is the stability of the analyte between the time of collection and the time of analysis. For many materials, including most of the commoner assays, this is not a problem, and the analyte is stable for days or even weeks unless the conditions for storage or transport are particularly extreme. However, there are some materials (Table 7.5) which are rapidly degraded by endogenous enzymes in serum or plasma unless steps are taken to prevent this. The principle means for obviating this problem are immediate separation of the plasma in a refrigerated centrifuge, following which the plasma is frozen and kept at $-20°C$ or lower throughout storage and transport and allowed to thaw only on the day of assay. An

TABLE 7.5

Examples of analytes which are liable to enzyme degradation in plasma or serum and should therefore be collected in the presence of enzyme inhibitors (Trasylol, 1000 KIU/ml; Zyznar, 1981) and kept deep-frozen during storage and transport

---

Corticotrophin (ACTH) and other ACTH –LPH-related peptides
Releasing hormones (e.g., gonadotrophin-releasing hormone, thyrotrophin-releasing hormone)
Arginine vasopressin (antidiuretic hormone)
Glucagon
Gastrin
Vasoactive intestinal peptide (VIP)
Parathyroid hormone
Calcitonin
Cyclic AMP
Vitamin D
Renin activity
Angiotensin
Prostaglandins

---

alternative, applicable to some but not all assays, is the inclusion of a potent enzyme inhibitor in the sample collection tube, or of ascorbate or 0.1% sodium azide in the case of serum folate. Even for those analytes which are considered to be very stable there are certain general points which can be made about sample storage and transport:

(1) Stability should always be tested and not assumed. A material which is unaffected by several days in the postal system of a country with a northern climate may behave quite differently under warmer conditions.

(2) The shortest possible time gap between sample collection and analysis is always desirable, both from the point of view of service to the patient and to avoid minor degrees of analyte degradation which may not be obvious even in carefully designed experiments.

(3) If there is any significant delay in the analysis of the sample (e.g., one week or longer) it should be stored deep-frozen. As always, repeated freezing and thawing should be avoided.

(4) It is usually assumed that identical results will be obtained on either serum or plasma, with the exception of assays for coagulation factors. However, significant differences have been demonstrated even with common assays such as thyroxine and cortisol (Kubasik and Sine, 1978); for this reason the type of sample should always be specified, and possible differences subject to rigorous experiment during development of the assay.

(5) The type of anticoagulant (e.g., heparin, EDTA–citrate) and tube (plastic, glass), should be specified and previously investigated.

A special problem of sample collection occurs with screening for congenital hypothyroidism in the neonate, a situation in which the amount of blood available may be very small. This has been successfully overcome by the development of assays for T4 and TSH which can be applied to dried blood spots on filter paper, a similar specimen to that collected for the Guthrie test (Larson and Broskin, 1975; Beckers et al., 1978).

CHAPTER 8

Requirements for binding assays – calculation of results

More effort is often devoted to complex methods for the calculation of results than to the equally important activities of optimising assay design and quality control systems. In this section are discussed both simple calculation and the more sophisticated data transformations which can be used with a calculator or computer to generate results automatically.

8.1. Calculation of results by manual extrapolation

Throughout the world the vast majority of binding assay results are calculated by this means. The standard points are plotted in any of the formats already described in § 1.6, and the points are then joined either by straight lines from one to the next or, more commonly, as the freehand curve which appears to the operator to most satisfactorily fit all the points. For those with an unsteady hand this procedure is facilitated by the use of a flexible ruler. The value of the bound/free distribution for an unknown sample is then located on this curve, and the corresponding standard value read from the horizontal axis (see Fig. 1.4). Any corrections for recovery of an extraction technique are applied to this value.

Several criticisms can be levelled at this procedure:

(1) Joining the points of the standard curve by straight lines may often yield an irregular 'curve' influenced by the errors of each individual point. This method is not recommended. Joining the points by a continuous 'line of best fit' as judged by eye is easily attacked because of the subjective nature of the operation. Nevertheless, the human eye and brain as an analog machine is greatly under-rated, and the end result will often be superior to that obtained by all but the most elaborate of electronic equipment. In particular, the eye

is capable of taking in and excluding error points which are obvious outliers and of forming curves which mathematically are highly complex.

(2) A much more important disadvantage of manual plotting and reading of results is the errors to which it may give rise. In one study (Jeffcoate and Das, 1977), in which raw count data from a specimen assay were sent to 35 different laboratories, manual calculation was found to be 4–7-times more variable than an automated method based on a logit–log fit. The errors include the straightforward mistake, when one of the co-ordinates is incorrectly read – a surprisingly common fault, especially if large series of figures are examined at one time. Errors also include variations in the manual drawing of a curve, and the tendency of many operators to round off figures to the nearest convenient integer – for example, to the nearest ten. These problems in manual calculation are much the best argument for machine calculation of results.

8.2. Data transformation of the standard curve

A wide variety of curve-fitting procedures is now available which permit on- or off-line calculation of results using a calculator or computer. These procedures can be divided into 'model-based' methods, which make assumptions about the underlying nature of the system, and 'data-based' methods which make no such assumptions (Table 8.1). The following generalisations can be made about these methods:

(1) It is likely that only the more complex methods will prove universally satisfactory;

(2) Model-based techniques are more efficient than data-based techniques in rejecting outliers (see § 8.4);

(3) Data-based methods are relatively simple to compute but require an extensive program for automatic assessment of 'goodness of fit'; they are also more likely than the model-based methods to accept 'garbage' which is mathematically correct but bears no relation to the underlying system;

(4) The 'spline' fits, which divide the standard curve into two parts, are only valid if an adequate number of standard points are available.

TABLE 8.1

Curve-fitting methods for binding assay data

These are divided into 'model-based' methods, which make assumptions about the underlying nature of the system, and 'data-based' methods which make no such assumptions. They are shown in increasing order of complexity which also corresponds, roughly, to the sequence of their introduction. The table is modified from Malan et al. (1978)

Model-based methods	Data-based methods
Dilution model (Hales and Randle, 1963)	Manual or polynomial curve-fits
Law of Mass Action (LMA) model (Meinert and McHugh, 1968; Chard, 1971)	Linear (polygonal) interpolation between points (Challand et al., 1976)
Logit–log model (Rodbard and Lewald, 1970)	Polynomial interpolation (Challand et al., 1976)
Logistic 4-parameter model (Healy, 1972; Rodbard and Hutt, 1974)	Spline fits (Marschner et al., 1973)
LMA 4-parameter model (Wilkins et al., 1978)	
Multiple binding site LMA model (Malan et al., 1978)	

Six is the absolute minimum; good results may only be expected with 10 or more points;

(5) No method is perfect, though at the present time the best is probably the logit transformation with the addition of one further parameter for asymmetry.

8.3. The logit transformation

The most familiar of the computation techniques is the 'logit transformation' introduced by Rodbard and Lewald (1970). Though not often realised, this is mathematically, identical to the mass-action equations given in § 1.7 and § 1.8. The logit is calculated as:

$$\text{logit } b = \log_e \left(\frac{b}{100-b} \right)$$

where b is the proportion of tracer bound expressed as a percentage of that in the zero standard. Plotted against log dose this yields a straight line for many if not all assays (see Fig. 1.14). This can be plotted manually (logit–log graph paper is available) but is readily adaptable to the linear regression programmes of simple calculators or computers and so allows automatic calculation of results using widely available hardware. However, certain practical points should be noted about the use of logit transformation:

(1) The assay blank value must be subtracted from the % bound before the logit is calculated. Failure to do this will yield a non-linear response. For the same reason, assays with a high and variable blank value are often poorly suited for logit transformation.

(2) The upper and lower 10% of a standard curve are frequently non-linear in logit-transformation and therefore should be eliminated when the line of best fit is drawn or calculated. Similarly, values recorded for unknowns above and below these limits should be rejected as inaccurate. Exclusion of values of this type is anyway good practice in a binding assay.

(3) The 'goodness of fit' of the straight line resulting from logit transformation is judged by the correlation coefficient or r value of a linear regression. It should be noted that, for a set of figures which the eye would consider a good fit, the r value is always 0.99 or greater. Lower figures imply a deviation from linearity or that one or more points are grossly in error.

(4) In some systems the logit transformation does not yield a straight line due to heterogeneity of the antiserum (see § 1.7). Usually this can be overcome by the use of an additional parameter for asymmetry, allowing the curve to approach its lower limit more slowly than its upper limit.

(5) The variable precision at different parts of the response (referred to as 'heteroscedasticity') implies that the best linearisation can only be obtained after weighting of the individual points; this procedure requires substantial computing facilities, though a simple manual alternative is to count each of the central points of the curve twice when performing the linear interpolation.

(6) The validity of the logit transformation is very dependent on good estimation of the '0' standard and the assay blank. Systems have been described in which these 'end parameters' can be adjusted as part of the line-fitting program (Healy, 1972; Hatch et al., 1979).

8.4. Identification of outliers

An 'outlier' is a result which appears to be uncharacteristic of a given assay system: for example, replicates of a sample or standard which show a difference much wider than that of other points in the system. Outliers can occur for two reasons;

(1) They may be due to a specific error in a given tube, such as failure to add one of the reagents;

(2) They may result from the simple statistical premise that in a variable system some points will vary more than others.

Methods for identifying and eliminating outliers are unsatisfactory. A sophisticated approach would be to compute the 'variation of the variation' for all points in a given assay run, and to eliminate those which lay outside a pre-determined statistical limit (e.g., where duplicates differ by more than twice the mean difference). This would be time-consuming in the absence of computational facilities. More common is to set an arbitrary upper limit, such as 5% in cases where the response is recorded as the percentage bound, or a fixed number of counts where this is used as the response metameter.

Neither approach is helpful when both of a pair of replicates are outliers with only a small difference between them. In the case of a sample assayed once at a single dose level this error is irretrievable. In the case of a point on a standard curve the deviation may be apparent because the mean of the point is not a good fit to the remainder of the curve (Fig. 8.1). The human eye and the more complex computer routines can take this into account but a special problem arises if the 'double outlier' is at one extreme of a standard curve; when this is atypical it may not be obvious to eye or machine but can have a disproportionate effect on the positioning of the curve (Fig. 8.1).

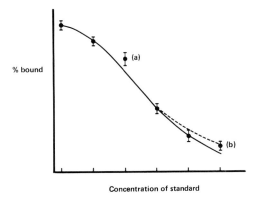

Fig. 8.1. Diagrammatic illustration of the problem of plotting a standard curve in the presence of outliers. Point (a) is a fairly obvious outlier: as it lies in the mid-section of the standard curve it is immediately apparent that it deviates from the line of best-fit to the remaining points; both the human eye or a well-controlled machine programme would eliminate this point. Point (b) is at an extreme of the standard curve and is therefore much more problematic. It would be difficult for the eye or a machine to determine whether point (b) or the preceding point is in error, and thus to judge between the continuous line or the interrupted line as the best description of the lower part of the standard curve.

8.5. *Estimation of confidence limits to the result of an unknown*

Every estimation has an error, and the purist would demand that this be presented as part of the result. In other words, that a value be not given simply as '10' but rather as '9–11'. A simple way to calculate this is to apply the within-assay error to the figure obtained. For example, if the coefficient of variation is known to be 5% then 95% limits to an estimate can be given as the observed value ± 10%.

It could be argued that the correct parameter to use is between-assay variation rather than within-assay variation. Thus, it is not only the individual result on one day which matters, but also how the result relates to a normal range which will have been generated from multiple assays. The problem with this approach is that the resulting confidence limits may appear almost ridiculously wide. For example, in a study of 17 laboratories in the UK (Jeffcoate, 1978), between-assay variation for prolactin ranged from 11.3–59.3%. A laboratory with a variation of 30% would have to report a result of '10' as '4–16'!

For a binding assay, estimation of confidence limits presents the problem of the variation of precision with dose (see § 11.2.1.5). Sophisticated approaches to the determination of error have been described (see Rodbard, 1971) using weighted values to take into account this variation but the procedure demands fairly elaborate computational facilities. Furthermore, because duplicates are subject to a large random sampling error, only limited statistical tests can be applied to a single dose level of the test sample. Finally, and most important, the majority of binding assays are performed as a clinical service and the average physician will not take kindly to receiving results as a range rather than a single figure. Calculation of error, other than as part of the quality control procedures which should be a feature of every assay (see Ch. 11), is unnecessary for most practical purposes.

8.6. *Electronic aids to calculation of results**

Virtually no laboratory today lacks some form of computational aid, even if it is only a simple calculator to work out means of replicates and percentages. More advanced aids to calculation can be divided into:

(1) The large general purpose calculator, such as the Hewlett Packard Model 10;

(2) The general purpose digital computer which can be of any size from 'micro' upwards;

(3) The 'dedicated' microprocessor, designed exclusively for the analysis of binding assay data and incorporated into the counter itself.

In turn, there are three ways in which any of these may be fed with the output of the counter:

* Useful reviews of automated calculation are G.S. Challand (ed.) (1978) Ann. Clin. Biochem. 15, 123, and pp. 373-614 of 'Radioimmunoassay and Related Procedures in Medicine, 1977', International Atomic Energy Agency, Vienna

(1) Manual introduction of figures read from the scaler or counter-printout;

(2) Use of punched tape output from the counter, which is then introduced via a tape-reader;

(3) A direct on-line connection to the counter.

The computer can produce a detailed analysis of the assay and its results in a neatly typed format. The calculator is more limited in its capabilities, particularly formatted output, but being relatively inexpensive is more likely to be available in the assay laboratory. Current developments in inexpensive microcomputers will probably make these the system of choice in the future, with the exception of those who have time-sharing access to a larger machine.

The type of input is again determined by availability. With a calculator the count data can be entered manually, but this is liable to error and punched tape is preferable. The large computer will almost always be fed with paper tape. Both can, in principle, operate directly on-line to the counter; however, this is wasteful because the slow rate of data entry, given the counting times currently in use, means that the data processor will only be operating at 1% or less of its potential speed unless it is linked to a group of counters or associated with the type of multi-detector counter which is becoming increasingly popular. Furthermore, some of the existing software packages are inflexible and have been criticised in routine clinical use (Logue et al., 1978). The best package should offer the user several options from the methods shown in Table 8.1; the type of machine and input will be determined by availability and practical necessity. The laboratory which conducts assays on only a few dozen samples weekly will probably use simple manual plotting. However, above a certain limit — probably around 20 samples in a single assay — machine calculation becomes both more efficient (because it eliminates errors) and cost-effective (because it saves operator time). For most laboratories the decision will anyway be pre-empted by the rapid introduction of multi-detector systems with in-built computational facilities.

CHAPTER 9

Characteristics of binding assays – sensitivity

9.1. Definition of sensitivity

Sensitivity is defined as the 'minimal detection limit of an assay'. Sometimes it is incorrectly used to describe other aspects such as the slope of the standard curve. 'Minimal detection limit' requires careful definition inasmuch as it is often judged from a cursory and over-optimistic inspection of the results of a single experiment. Rather, it should refer to the least concentration of unlabelled ligand which can be distinguished from a sample containing no unlabelled ligand, the distinction being based on the confidence limits of the estimate of the zero standard on the one hand and the standard on the other. This concept is illustrated in Fig. 9.1. Furthermore, confidence limits in this context should be described as a statistical function and not merely as the mean and range of a pair of replicates. For example, consider a pair of estimates of 100 and 105 (which could be any parameter reflecting the response in the standard curve); this would yield a mean of 102.5 with confidence limits of 97.6–107.4. If further replicates are available the confidence limits are sharply reduced. Thus, the set of estimates 99, 100, 105 and 106, which has the same mean but an apparently broader range, gives confidence limits of 99.1–105.9.

An alternative but less satisfactory way of defining sensitivity is as some arbitrary decrease from the '0' standard – for example, a 10% fall in relative binding. This may be useful as a rule of thumb for assays with '0' standard binding of greater than 40%, but for the reasons shown in Fig. 9.4 it is not appropriate for systems with lower levels of '0' binding.

A practical point of vital importance becomes obvious from Fig. 9.1 and the discussion above. It is that the minimal detection limit of an assay is critically dependent on the precision of the assay. Great efforts to

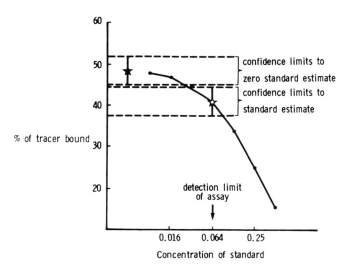

Fig. 9.1. The definition of 'sensitivity' or 'minimal detection limits' of an assay. This is the least quantity of ligand which can be distinguished from a sample containing no ligand (the zero standard). Note that this figure is critically dependent on the precision with which the estimates are made.

optimise assay design, on the lines set out below, will be completely vitiated if the reproducibility of estimates is poor. A further point which emerges, and which is rarely taken into account in the literature, is that the minimal detection limits are likely to vary from one assay to the next and from one operator to another. Thus, a lower limit stated as '10' on the basis set out above will not apply to an individual assay in which the replication of this point or the zero standard, or both, is poor. Under these circumstances the lower limit might become 20 or even 40.

A final point in the definition of sensitivity is the units in which it is specified. This should always be in terms of concentration (i.e., weight/ volume), and should refer to the biological fluid for which the assay is intended. A common fault is to specify the absolute amount of ligand in a given tube rather than its concentration: suppose an assay has a true sensitivity of 1 ng/ml; for an incubation volume of 1 ml this gives an absolute quantity of 1 ng; for a volume of 0.1 ml it gives 0.1 ng. To the unwary the latter would appear to be the more sensitive, but in reality they are identical. Another fault is to specify sensitivity with respect to standard in aqueous buffer solution, and this may not apply to a biological sample. Thus, sensitivity should always be expressed as the *concentration* in the *biological fluid* under investigation.

Extreme sensitivity is often regarded as the hallmark of a good assay. This arises from the fact that when radioimmunoassay was first introduced it was the sensitivity of the procedure, relative to other techniques, which led to its rapid establishment in biology and medicine. Yet for many important compounds high sensitivity is not a requirement since the levels in biological fluids are orders of magnitude above the minimal detection limits of the assay. There is much to be said for adjusting the conditions of the assay in such a way that the standard curve corresponds to the range of biological interest, assuming no sample dilution. 'Biological targeting' of this type is usually more important than maximisation of sensitivity.

9.2. *Methods of increasing the sensitivity of a binding assay*

The choice of reagent concentrations in a binding assay has already been described briefly (see § 1.5), and in this section the conditions for achieving maximum sensitivity will be discussed in more detail. Several approaches may be combined in any one assay.

9.2.1. *Reducing the amount of tracer*

This is the most familiar approach and is highly effective provided that its limitations are recognised. Unfortunately, there is a widespread assumption that the minimal detection limits of an assay are directly related to the amount of tracer used; in other words, that the sensitivity of an assay can be increased indefinitely simply by reducing the amount of tracer. This assumption, in turn, has led to the pursuit of high specific activity tracers, with all their attendant problems, when in reality a tracer of much lower activity would be perfectly adequate.

The limitations on the amount of tracer can be judged both from theoretical analysis (see § 1.8 and 1.9) and by experiment. The conclusions of either approach can be summarised as follows: that for any given set of conditions (affinity and concentration of binder, time of incubation, etc.) there is a limiting concentration of tracer below which further reduction leads to no significant change in the position of the standard curve or the sensitivity of the assay.

This concept is illustrated in Fig. 9.2. In practice, an approach to finding the appropriate concentration of tracer for use in an assay is as follows:

(1) Select, as a rule of thumb, a concentration of tracer approximately equivalent to the least amount of unlabelled ligand which the assay is intended to measure;

(2) Perform a binder dilution curve and select the concentration of antibody which binds around 50% of the tracer;

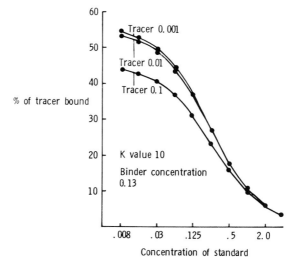

Fig. 9.2. Increasing the sensitivity of a binding assay by decreasing the amount of tracer (theoretical system, see § 1.8). Note that below a certain limiting level (0.01 in this case) further reduction in tracer does not alter the characteristics of the assay.

(3) Set up standard curves using this antibody concentration but with three different concentrations of tracer – the amount specified under (1) above, an amount one-tenth of this, and an amount ten times this value.

The result, if the antiserum has adequate affinity, will be three standard curves which can be interpreted as shown in Fig. 9.2. Other experimental approaches to the choice of a lower limit of tracer concentration have been described: for example, preparing a set of binder dilution curves with different amounts of tracer or a mixture of tracer and unlabelled ligand, or selecting a fixed concentration of standard at the intended limit of the assay and then comparing this with the zero standard using different amounts of tracer.

The choice of the optimal amount of tracer has implications for the initial preparation of labelled ligand. In operative terms the aim is a tracer yielding total counts of 10,000 in 1 min or less. If the least amount of tracer dictated by the above experiments yields considerably more counts, then it should be possible to reduce the specific activity of the initial preparation with all the advantages (less damage, easier handling) attendant upon this. Equally, the experiments might dictate an increase in specific activity.

9.2.2. Improving the quality of tracer

Making a better tracer can sometimes yield dramatic improvement in the sensitivity of an assay. To take an extreme example, if a tracer contained 50% of damaged components then the conditions selected for the assay (based on the 50% rule, see § 9.2.1) might yield '0' standard binding of 25%. Further purification to eliminate the damaged components would raise this figure to 50%, and the resulting increase in precision could increase the sensitivity 2-fold or more. The extent to which quality of tracer can affect sensitivity depends to some extent on the characteristics of the separation procedure (see § 6.1). If the separation can distinguish between damaged and undamaged tracer (i.e., the damaged tracer is selectively removed), then the quality of the tracer is relatively unimportant.

9.2.3. Reducing the amount of binder

Reducing the amount of binder will increase the sensitivity of an assay. Inspection of a theoretical example (Fig. 9.3) might suggest that there is no limit to the increase, but in practice it is constrained by the precision of the assay. Take, for example, a curve with a zero standard of only 10%. When this is drawn out on the scale shown in Fig. 9.4 it might at first sight seem to offer exceptional sensitivity. But when the confidence limits of the replicates are taken into account it can be seen that the first point which differs significantly from the zero standard is almost in the middle of the curve. With meticulous attention to detail, and particularly to the reduction of the assay blank values to less than 1%, it is possible to achieve optimal sensitivity and precision with a zero standard of this order (Wide, 1978). However, increasing sensitivity by decreasing the binder must always be a balance between what can be achieved theoretically and the reproducibility of replicates within the assay. As a rule of thumb, the use of conditions in which the zero standard is 20% or less of the total counts is often counter-productive — any increase in apparent sensitivity being negated by the decrease in precision.

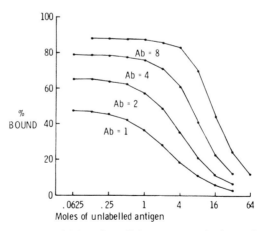

Fig. 9.3. Increasing the sensitivity of a radioimmunoassay by decreasing the amount of antibody (theoretical system, see § 1.9). Note that reducing the amount of antibody progressively increases the sensitivity, though this is eventually limited by the precision of estimates at the individual points.

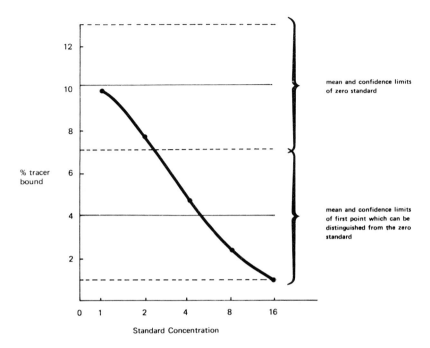

Fig. 9.4. How an apparently very sensitive assay, based on the use of a low concentration of binder (10% bound in the zero standard) is in reality much less sensitive because of the wide confidence limits to individual points.

9.2.4. Increasing the incubation time

Increasing the incubation time is not, in itself, a means of increasing sensitivity. However, it may be implicit in the use of very low concentrations of reagents which will require a considerable length of time to reach equilibrium. In exploring the lower limits of an assay, total incubation times of up to 7 days may be necessary. It might be assumed that antibodies of high K-value (i.e., with a large k_1) would come to equilibrium very rapidly. However, there is evidence with multivalent antigens and antibodies that some conformations affording thermodynamically very stable binding are only rarely obtained (Barisas et al., 1977), and attainment of true equilibrium may be very slow indeed. This is due to the fact that the most favourable free energy may only be achieved when the highly flexible antibody molecule passes through an infrequently attained conformation.

Apart from achieving equilibrium with low concentrations of reagents, lengthy incubation times have almost no advantages and several disadvantages. Thus, they expose the reagents, and in particular the tracer, to the risk of damage by other components of the assay system: for example, in the case of protein hormones, to attack by proteolytic enzymes. For this reason it is often found that binding in the zero standard shows a progressive decrease with increasing incubation time, a point which is clearly unfavourable in terms of sensitivity. Furthermore, long incubation periods are technically inconvenient: storage space is required for large numbers of tubes; errors due to tube misclassification become more likely; and there is a substantial delay in the reporting of results to the clinician. In the initial development of an assay every effort should be made to *reduce the incubation time*.

9.2.5. Reducing the incubation time – disequilibrium assays

If an assay is interrupted by separation of bound and free ligand before equilibrium is reached then zero standard binding is reduced and the apparent sensitivity may be increased. The effect is not dissimilar to that obtained by reduction in the concentration of antibody, the main difference being that it is achieved more rapidly. However, the separation procedure takes a finite length of time. If this is a significant fraction of the total time taken for the assay, then the possibility arises of a substantial difference between the first and last tubes of a run, the last tube having had rather more time to reach equilibrium. An approach of this type requires great attention to detail if it is to be successful.

Dramatic reductions in incubation time are now becoming the hallmark of many radioimmunoassay kits. Sometimes it is achieved at the expense of a loss of accuracy; for example, in a survey of serum gastrin kits, substantial deviations from a reference method were noted with incubation periods of 1.5–3 h, which could be corrected by extending the time to 24 h (Gibson et al., 1977). Assays with unusually short incubation times should be carefully evaluated for this phenomenon.

9.2.6. Order of addition of reagents

The usual order of addition of reagents in a binding assay is sample—tracer—binder, and both unlabelled and labelled ligand have equal access to the binding sites. However, if the order of addition of tracer and binder is reversed (i.e., sample—binder—tracer) the end-result can be a standard curve with much improved sensitivity (Samols and Bilkus, 1963). This is the so-called 'late-addition' assay and the effect has been attributed to the formation of multivalent antigen—antibody complexes which are less likely to dissociate than univalent complexes (Ichihara et al., 1979). An example is shown in Fig. 9.5. Assays for low M_r antigens (e.g., haptens) usually do not show this effect because they cannot form multivalent complexes.

9.2.7. Purification of binder

Antisera usually contain antibody populations of different affinities and superficially it might appear desirable to select only those of highest

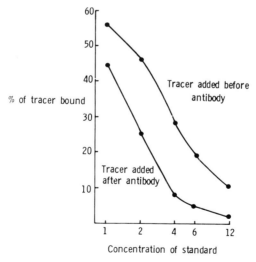

Fig. 9.5. Increasing the sensitivity of a radioimmunoassay by adding the tracer after, rather than before, the antibody (radioimmunoassay for human placental lactogen).

affinity. This can be achieved by prior treatment of the antiserum with an immunoadsorbent, low affinity antibody molecules being eluted using mild dissociating conditions, and higher affinity molecules with more drastic conditions (Massaglia et al., 1974). Purification of an antiserum in this manner has several potential technical disadvantages: it would require a substantial supply of pure antigen for the preparation of the immunosorbent; it would be wasteful of antiserum because of poor recoveries; it would be time-consuming and technically demanding; and it could result in damage to the antibody under the conditions used for dissociation of the molecules of highest affinity. More important, it is doubtful if the intended effect is ever actually achieved. On theoretical grounds, simple dilution of an antiserum constitutes an immunopurification, since at low concentrations only those molecules of high affinity will be significantly involved in the antibody—antigen reaction. A possible exception to this would be if the antibody population consisted of a very small number of high affinity molecules and a very large number of low affinity molecules. Finally, it has never been convincingly demonstrated in practice that antibody selection yields an increase in sensitivity. Thus, purification of antibody cannot be recommended as a routine procedure, though it is, of course, an essential part of immunometric techniques (see § 6.4).

A variant on the purification of antibody is the use of a 'stripping' procedure (see § 2.2) to remove endogenous ligand from the antisera (Kruse, 1979). For example, an antiserum to thyroxine (T4) will itself contain the animal's own endogenous T4 which will be bound to the antibody sites of highest affinity – thus effectively blocking them.

9.2.8. Increasing the sample volume

Sensitivity can be increased by an increase in sample volume relative to the other components of the assay. In many assays the sample represents only 10% of the total incubation mixture (e.g., 50 μl in 0.5 ml); yet the other reagents could be added in as little as 50 μl and at first sight there would seem to be no objection to increasing the sample volume to 450 μl, thus enhancing sensitivity 9-fold. In practice, this approach is limited by the fact that biological fluids will often produce non-specific interference if incorporated at high concentrations (see § 10.3). The degree of interference varies considerably with the separation system, and is probably least with well-optimised second-antibody and solid-phase systems. As a rule of thumb (but with several exceptions) non-specificity due to irrelevant materials in the sample is insignificant if the total concentration of sample in the incubation mixture does not exceed 10%.

9.2.9. Temperature of incubation

The rate of approach to equilibrium of a binding assay will approximately double for every 10°C rise in temperature. This principle may be used to enhance the speed of an assay; however, it will not usually affect sensitivity, and will increase the rate of undesirable reactions such as enzymic destruction of the tracer. In practice the upper limit of temperature is 45°C. With assays which use a circulating binding protein, the affinity constant and sensitivity are substantially increased at lower temperatures. Immunoassays for steroids may show a similar phenomenon, and if extreme sensitivity is required the use of low temperatures should be explored (Keane et al., 1976).

An assay which is temperature-dependent can present serious practical problems. Maintenance of large numbers of tubes at a fixed and identical temperature is not simple; if a rack of closely packed tubes is removed from a refrigerator and placed on the laboratory bench a significant temperature difference (5°C or more) can soon develop between tubes on the periphery of the rack and those in the centre.

9.2.10. Increasing the number of replicates

It has already been emphasised that sensitivity is critically dependent on precision. In turn, the confidence limits to an estimate are dependent on the number of replicate determinations; increasing this number will narrow the confidence limits and thus enhance the sensitivity of the assay. This approach is little used in practice because of the extra work involved. Nevertheless, of all methods so far discussed, it is the only one which for a given set of reagents and conditions produces an almost unlimited increase in sensitivity.

9.2.11. Extraction and concentration

The means by which sensitivity can be enhanced by extraction and concentration have already been described in § 7.1.

9.2.12. Immunometric assays

It has often been emphasised that immunometric assays (§ 6.4) are capable of greater sensitivity than conventional techniques (Ekins, 1980). If the labelled antibody is used in excess then sensitivity is less dependent on affinity and more on classical considerations of signal-to-noise ratio, e.g., the least amount of radioactivity which can be detected above background. This principle has not, as yet, been widely applied in practical assays.

9.3. Methods of decreasing the sensitivity of an assay – increasing the antibody concentration

The importance of targeting the standard curve to a range of clinical and biological interest has already been described. Most radioimmunoassays have a potential sensitivity which is considerably in excess of that required for routine operation, and it is thus a positive advantage to decrease the sensitivity.

The primary method for decreasing sensitivity is to increase the concentration of the binder. This will yield a progressive shift of the standard curve towards higher concentrations of unlabelled ligand (Fig. 9.6). An increase in binder concentration has several implications for the operation of an assay which can be summarised as follows:

(1) *Concentration of tracer*:   When the binder concentration is increased the amount of tracer can also be increased with a corresponding decrease in the counting time required. Furthermore, the specific activity of the tracer can be reduced with all that this implies in terms of 'damage' and increased stability. In a grossly desensitised assay, such as that shown in Fig. 9.6, a very low specific activity tracer can be used in sufficient quantity to yield adequate counts in 10 sec or less, with no detriment to the position or shape of the standard curve.

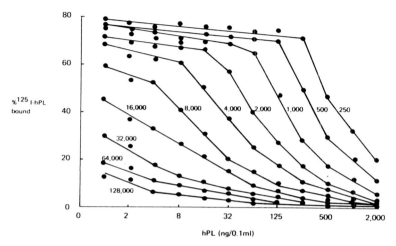

Fig. 9.6. Desensitisation of a radioimmunoassay for human placental lactogen. Increasing concentration of antibody (shown as the reciprocal of the titre at which it is used) produces a progressive shift of the standard curve to the right.

(2) *Zero standard and shape of curve*:   The use of a large amount of binder implies a high level of binding in the 'zero' standard; following from this the curve will be steeper, and estimates of unknowns are more precise.

(3) *Incubation time*:   The use of high concentrations of all reagents means that equilibrium is reached very rapidly. For an extreme example such as that of Fig. 9.6, at higher concentrations of antiserum equilibrium is virtually instantaneous, and the separating agent can be added immediately after the binder.

(4) *Sample volume*:   With a desensitised assay there is no need for prior dilution of the sample, thus eliminating a source of error. Small volumes can be used (in practice, as little as 10 μl) which reduces non-specific effects and requires only a small specimen of blood from the patient. This is of particular importance today when multiple tests on a single sample are becoming the rule rather than the exception.

(5) *Affinity of the binder*:   If the binder is used in relative excess it does not have to be of exceptionally high affinity. Thus, an antiserum rejected because it will not yield a certain level of sensitivity may be perfectly satisfactory for an assay targeted to a lower sensitivity.

(6) *Supply of binder*:   Desensitised assays using high concentrations of binder will place considerable demands on its supply. One ml of an antiserum used at 1:100,000 will suffice for the assay of some 40,000 samples; the same amount of antiserum used at 1:1,000 is only enough for 400 samples.

(7) *Convenience*:   Most of the features set out above – short incubation times, short counting times, optimal shape of standard curve – make for technical convenience in the performance of the assay. It cannot be reiterated often enough that the eventual clinical value of a technique is directly and completely related to the ease, speed and reliability with which it is carried out.

(8) *'Early addition' of tracer*:   The sensitivity of an assay can also be reduced by adding the tracer before the unlabelled ligand (this is the reverse of 'late addition' of tracer which increases the sensitivity, see § 9.2.6). Where applicable this yields a very simple assay: the sample is added to a single pre-formed tracer–antibody complex (usually solid-phase) and the amount of radioactivity released is a measure of the unlabelled ligand present (Weetall and Odstrchel, 1976; Cocola et al., 1979).

9.4. *Targeting of binding assays – the importance of ranges*

An assay should be arranged to suit a clinical purpose, rather than vice-versa. The basic principle is that the most precise part of the standard curve (usually the central portion) should be set so that it coincides with the range of practical interest: this may either be the whole of a normal range (for materials with which both high and low values may be of diagnostic significance) or one extreme of a normal range (for materials

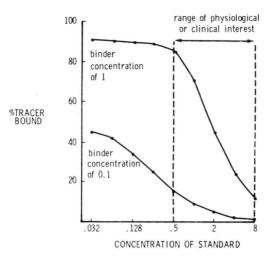

Fig. 9.7. Targeting a binding assay by varying the concentration of binder. A very sensitive assay is yielded by a binder concentration of 0.1, but, it embraces only part of the range of physiological or clinical interest. By increasing the binder concentration to 1, a less sensitive standard curve is produced which covers the range of interest and is also considerably steeper.

with which either low values or high values but not both, are of diagnostic significance). The principle is illustrated in Fig. 9.7 and 9.8.

9.5. Optimisation of an assay by theoretical analysis

If a binder–ligand system can be fully characterised with respect to the absolute concentrations of reactants, the K-value of the binder and the errors implicit in the determination of the distribution of bound and free ligand, then it is possible to substitute these factors in a theoretical model and thus, by a purely mathematical exercise, to explore the performance of the assay and to select optimal concentrations of reagents. The simplest model is the algebraic expression of the mass action equation set out in § 1.8 and eq. (16). However, this takes no account of factors such as differences between tracer and unlabelled ligand, hetero-

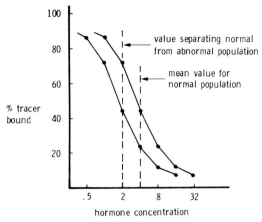

Fig. 9.8. Targeting of a binding assay. If the aim is to study a normal population, then the mid-point of the standard curve should be chosen as the mean value of the normal population (curve on right). If the aim is separation of a normal from an abnormal population, then the mid-point should be the value which best separates these two populations (curve on left).

geneity of the binder, and errors in determination. Vastly more sophistic-ated techniques have been described which take these factors into ac-count: all require the use of a computer, together with a degree of ma-thematical understanding which is exceptional in most workers in the biomedical field. Excellent reviews of this area are available (e.g., Ekins, 1974). However, simple experimental trial and error on the lines set out above can often yield equally satisfactory answers.

9.6. Conclusions

Optimisation of assay design is at the very core of radioimmunoassay and related techniques. All other aspects — preparation and examination of reagents — are in reality only branches of chemistry and biochemistry. The points emphasised in this chapter are the correct definition of sen-sitivity, the means for achieving the highest possible level of sensitivity, and, most important, the targeting of the assay with respect to its intend-ed use — the only merit of a technique being in its practical application.

CHAPTER 10

Characteristics of binding assays – specificity

10.1. Definition of specificity

The specificity of an assay can be defined as 'the degree to which an assay responds to substances other than that for which the assay was designed'. The extent to which a given compound can interfere with an assay is often referred to as 'cross-reaction' or 'potency'.

The subject of specificity will be discussed under the headings of 'specific non-specificity' and 'non-specific non-specificity'. The former refers to interference by identifiable materials which are physicochemically similar to the ligand and may thus react directly with the binder. The latter refers to interference by materials which do not directly react with the binder, but can nevertheless affect the primary binder–ligand reaction; for example, acid conditions which produce partial or total inhibition of any antigen–antibody reaction.

10.2. Specific non-specificity

There are many groups of biological materials which are physicochemically very similar; for example, the various steroid hormones, or the glycoprotein hormones of the anterior pituitary gland (LH, FSH, TSH). The specificity of their physiological action depends on target organ receptors capable of distinguishing between them on the basis of small differences in the molecule. The use of these receptors in binding assays confers similar specificity but is limited to those substances which have an effect on a target organ. For most purposes other types of binder are used and the discussion which follows will be devoted largely to antibodies.

10.2.1. The basis of specific non-specificity

An antiserum to a given material will usually react, albeit less effectively, with closely related materials. There are three reasons why this may occur:

(1) A single homogeneous antibody population may react with a range of related ligands, each reaction having a different affinity constant;

(2) The antiserum may contain populations of antibody molecules one or more of which is directed to a site on the primary material which also occurs on a related material;

(3) The antiserum may contain antibodies directed to contaminants present in the ligand and which are also present in the related material (Fig. 10.1).

These concepts are important to an understanding of the experimental finding of 'parallelism' or 'non-parallelism'. If the difference between two related materials is solely in their K-value with respect to a single homogeneous binder, then standard curves for these materials using a homologous tracer will be parallel. Exceptions to this may be seen if the tracer is not homologous and if the mass of tracer represents a significant fraction of the total ligand in a given tube. This type of non-parallelism is found only at the lowest concentrations of unlabelled ligand and would be barely apparent from simple inspection of a standard curve.

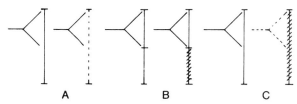

Fig. 10.1. Different types of specific non-specificity. (A) A single population of antibody molecules reacts with two related materials, but with a different affinity constant (i.e., one molecule is a good 'fit' to the combining site, the other is a less good fit). (B) A single population of antibody molecules reacts with an antigenic site which is held in common between two different molecules (e.g., the α-subunit of the glycoprotein hormones). (C) The antiserum contains populations of antibodies to different ligands; the non-specific ligand may then cross-react in the assay.

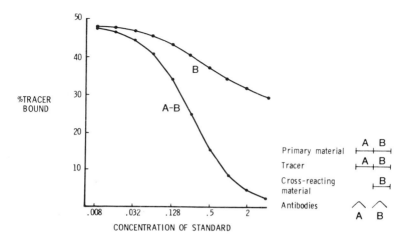

Fig. 10.2. Non-parallelism due to heterogeneity. The primary material and the tracer have two antigenic stites, A and B. The antiserum contains two corresponding populations of antibodies. Material containing site B only will produce the curve shown. It can never produce complete inhibition in the assay because antibodies of population A will always by unoccupied and can still bind the tracer.

The second and third types of non-specificity — due to heterogeneity of binder or binding sites — can yield more dramatic non-parallelism. The principle by which this can influence the shape of a standard curve is best illustrated by an extreme case (Fig. 10.2). Clearly, the precise result obtained will vary with the set of reagents used and, in the case of radioimmunoassay, the distribution of antibody populations will vary considerably between different antisera. One might yield apparent parallelism between two cross-reacting materials, while another would yield non-parallelism.

In a real system the three types of specific non-specificity may often co-exist. The analysis of the main factor involved — heterogeneity of K-value at a single site, or heterogeneity of sites — can then become very complex. However, gross non-parallelism suggests site heterogeneity, an observation of great practical importance because it indicates that specificity may be improved by absorption of the antiserum.

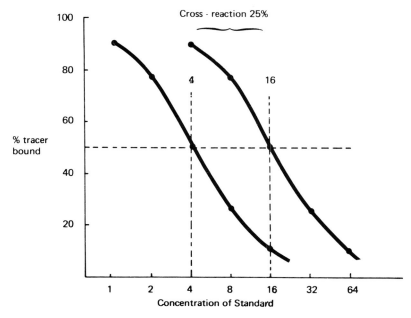

Fig. 10.3. Estimation of the percentage cross-reaction from the amounts of material required to produce 50% inhibition in the assay. The curve on the left is for the standard, that on the right for the cross-reacting material. Note that this procedure cannot be applied if the curves are non-parallel.

10.2.2. Assessment of specific non-specificity

To test specificity, serial dilutions of the material in question are prepared and assayed: the resulting curve is then compared with that given by the standard material for which the assay was designed. The commonest way of presenting the result is to compare the amount of the cross-reacting material which yields 50% inhibition of binding with the amount of standard giving the same inhibition, and then to express the potency of the material as a percentage of that of the standard (Fig. 10.3) (Abraham, 1969). For example, if the respective concentrations are 1 and 100, the potency is stated as 1%. Other methods of defining cross-reactions include comparison of the slopes of standard curves (Feldman et al., 1972), and comparison of the response to a fixed level of ligand (e.g., 1 ng) (Lauzon et al., 1972).

A number of aspects of the subject will be considered.

(1) *Concentration by weight versus molar concentration*:   Potency should always be calculated on the basis of molar concentrations rather than weight concentrations. For example, if the M_r-value of the cross-reacting material is 10 times that of the standard, and the potency by *weight* is given as 10%, then the two materials are equal on a molar basis.

(2) *Variation with conditions of assay*:   The apparent potency of a cross-reacting material may vary if the conditions of the assay are changed. For example, specificity can show great variation according to the nature of the tracer employed (Fig. 10.4).

(3) *Calculation if curves are non-parallel*:   If the curves yielded by standard and cross-reacting material are non-parallel, then clearly a calculation of potency made at 50% inhibition will be very different from that made at 10% (see Fig. 10.3). There is no simple answer to this problem, and non-parallel cross-reaction must be judged in relation to the intended clinical use of the assay, for example, by the use of a fixed arbitrary level (e.g., 1 ng) of the cross-reacting antigens.

Arising from this is the question of how to judge parallelism. A subjective impression can easily miss substantial differences, particularly at the extremes of the curve. There are two objective approaches:

(i) To perform a logit transformation of the results (see § 8.2), and compare the two linear regressions.

(ii) To calculate the apparent potency of each dilution, and then to examine the figures for any systematic deviation between standard and cross-reacting material.

In judging non-parallelism it is also important to exclude experimental artefact; for example, comparison of *serial* dilutions of a material with independently prepared dilutions of the same material is almost certain to yield some degree of non-parallelism. (see § 2.5).

(4) *Choice of materials to examine for cross-reaction*:   It is impossible to examine every conceivable biological material for cross-reaction in an as-

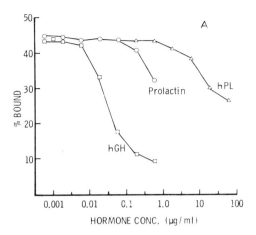

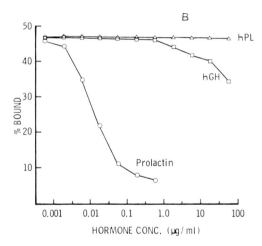

Fig. 10.4. Standard curves for human growth hormone (hGH), human prolactin, and human placental lactogen (hPL) using an antiserum to a partially purified preparation of human prolactin: (A) tracer is [125] I-labelled hGH; (B) tracer is [125] I-labelled prolactin. Note that the specificity of this assay is almost entirely dictated by the nature of the tracer. With appropriate choice of the latter, a relatively non-specific antibody can yield a highly specific assay. (From data kindly supplied by Dr. A.S. McNeilly.)

say. In practice, a judicious selection has to be made from those substances whose physicochemical nature suggests that cross-reaction is likely. With steroid hormones and small peptides, the choice is relatively easy since the different structures and their relationship are well-understood. However, with larger proteins the choice of materials may be considerably more difficult. Highly purified preparations are generally scarce and relatively large amounts may be needed to exclude cross-reaction at the 1% and 0.1% levels. The use of impure material can be misleading since this may contain related proteins which react in the assay, but do not feature in the definition of 'purity' derived from studies with another type of assay (see § 12.4). Finally, some substances are biologically unique and there is no logical basis for selecting other materials for specificity studies: specificity must then depend on the physicochemical characterisation of the substance, together with its apparent behaviour under physiological conditions.

(5) *Effect of primary antigen*:   Tests of cross-reaction are usually carried out in antigen-free fluid using only tracer amounts of the primary antigen. Yet an authentic sample may often contain substantial amounts of the primary antigen. It has been suggested that tests of specificity should be carried out both in the presence and absence of added primary antigen, and that the results of such tests may obviate the need for complex extraction procedures (Dotti et al., 1979).

(6) *Species specificity*:   Where a material is chemically identical in a wide range of different species (e.g., steroid hormones, thyroxine) a single assay is adequate for all studies. Where the material is not identical (e.g., most large protein hormones) species specificity has to be established by experiment. The results range from those with the pituitary glycoprotein hormones, with which there may be no cross-reaction whatever (Odell et al., 1967), to prolactin or parathormone with which the cross-reaction is sufficient to permit measurement of circulating levels in the human using materials of animal origin.

10.2.3. Relevance of specificity to physiological and clinical studies

The eventual significance of a cross-reacting material lies in the extent to which it is likely to interfere with the practical operation of an assay. This is illustrated by two extreme examples. Radioimmunoassays for thyroxine (T_4) often show a substantial cross-reaction (10% or more) with triiodothyronine (T_3); however, as the circulating levels of T_3 are at least two orders of magnitude lower than those of T_4 this cross-reaction is unimportant in practice. At the other extreme, a radioimmunoassay for T_3 may show a cross-reaction of 1% with T_4 which could be highly critical; with such an assay circulating T_4 would make a substantial contribution to the result.

Sometimes non-specificity of an assay can be a practical advantage. For example, a radioimmunoassay for nortryptiline may cross-react with a variety of other tricyclic antidepressant drugs; since administration of more than one of these at a time is rare, a single combination of antibody and tracer can, with the appropriate choice of standards, yield valid estimates for a wide range of materials (Aherne et al., 1977; Maguire et al., 1978).

10.2.4. Methods for improving specificity

With the naturally occurring binders (circulating proteins or cell receptors) there is little which can be done to alter the specificity of the assay itself, other than the use of the preliminary extraction procedures which have already been described (see § 7.2). With antibodies, by contrast, the variability and heterogeneity of the primary reagent offers many opportunities for the direct improvement of specificity. Potential approaches include the following.

10.2.4.1. Choice of immunogen   Non-specificity of type A (Fig. 10.1) (due to reaction of a single homogeneous antibody population with a range of related antigenic sites) can be influenced by the choice of immunogen, especially in the case of a hapten (§ 5.2.3). For example, specificity of an antibody to oestrogens will be largely determined by the very characteristic A ring. If the oestrogen is coupled to the carrier via the carbon-3 of the A ring most of this specificity will be lost: for this reason the immunogen is almost invariably prepared through the carbon-6 position.

Non-specificity of type B (due to the presence of common antigenic sites on the ligand and related material) can be avoided if the immunogen used is a fragment of the ligand which does not contain the common antigenic site. For example, the glycoprotein hormones (LH, FSH, TSH, hCG) each consists of two subunits: the α-subunit which is identical in all four; and the β-subunit which is different in all four and confers biological specificity. Because of the common α-subunit, assays based on intact hormone often show striking cross-reactions among all types, whereas, the use of β-subunit as immunogen and tracer yields an assay specific for the individual hormone. However, the isolated subunit may have a tertiary structure different from that in the intact molecule, and therefore a different antigenic structure. Assays based on this principle are sometimes less efficient, in terms of antibody affinity and sensitivity, than assays directed to the intact molecule. For example, the 'MB' isoenzyme of creatinine kinase, which contains equal numbers of M and B subunits, shows only limited cross-reaction in an assay specific to the B-subunit (Zweig et al., 1978).

Non-specificity of type C (due to the presence of irrelevant materials in the ligand) can be avoided if it is possible to use pure immunogen. For example, earlier problems with the specificity of antisera to pituitary glycoprotein hormones (LH, FSH, TSH) have been virtually overcome by the use of highly purified materials as immunogens (Thorell and Holmstron, 1976).

10.2.4.2. Manipulation of conditions of assay   The specificity of an assay may vary with the conditions chosen. For example, non-specificity due to a population of low affinity antibody molecules may become insignificant if the antiserum is used at very high dilutions. Non-specificity may also result from the use of short incubation disequilibrium assays; binding of a ligand and cross-reacting material may be virtually equivalent under these circumstances, and only at equilibrium does the relatively greater dissociation rate of the cross-reacting material yield a relative excess of bound primary ligand. It is essential for this reason to re-check the specificity of an antibody under the exact conditions used in the assay.

10.2.4.3. Removal of unwanted populations of antibody   Non-specificity of types B and C can be eliminated by prior absorption of the antiserum — in the case of type B with a purified preparation of a fragment of the molecule containing the common antigenic sequence; in the case of type

C with a preparation of the contaminant material. Sometimes the two approaches are combined. For example, in the earlier days of gonadotrophin assays it was customary to absorb antisera to hFSH with a preparation of hCG. This had two effects:

(1) To remove populations of antibodies directed to the common α-subunit;

(2) Because of the close similarity between LH and hCG, to remove populations of antibodies to LH resulting from LH as a contaminant in the FSH used as immunogen.

However, the gain in specificity was accompanied by a loss of sensitivity. Elimination of type B non-specificity by absorption can also be used to render an assay specific for a 'neo-antigen' — that is an antigen which is expressed in a fragment of the molecule but not, because of the differences in tertiary structure, in the intact molecule. This is well-illustrated by the assay of fibrinogen degradation products (Fig. 10.5). An antiserum to the terminal fragment D contains antibodies specific to the frag-

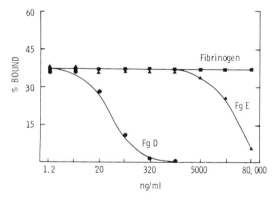

Fig. 10.5. Improving specificity by absorption of an antiserum. In this case the antiserum was raised to pure fragment D (FgD), one of the terminal degradation products of fibrinogen, and then absorbed with fibrinogen. Used with a tracer of ^{125}I-labelled fragment D this antiserum shows no cross-reaction with intact fibrinogen at the concentrations tested and relatively little cross-reaction with fragment E (FgE). Since fragment D is part of the fibrinogen molecule, this assay is specific to a 'neo-antigen', i.e. one that is revealed during the course of proteolytic destruction of fibrinogen. (From data kindly supplied by Dr. Y.B. Gordon.)

ment itself, and in addition antibodies which will react with intact fibrinogen. Absorption of the antiserum with fibrinogen removes the latter population and thus yields an assay specific for fragment D with no interference by the parent molecule.

In practical terms there are two approaches to the absorption of an antiserum:

(1) Simple addition of the cross-reacting material, and removal of the resulting immunoprecipitate by centrifugation. This has the disadvantage that soluble complexes may remain due to the 'prozone' phenomenon;

(2) Addition of the cross-reacting material in insoluble form, for example, in the case of a protein, after crosslinking with glutaraldehyde.

A more general technique is the use of antigen coupled to a solid phase (see Appendix VI). The solid phase can then be added batchwise to the antiserum, or used in the form of a column to which the antiserum is applied and then eluted.

10.2.4.4. Other methods of improving specificity

(1) *The separation technique for bound and free ligand*: For example, the cross-reaction of 5α-dihydrotestosterone in a testosterone assay is reduced if ammonium sulphate is used for separation rather than dextran-coated charcoal (Tyler et al., 1973). The mechanism of this phenomenon is uncertain.

(2) *Correction of results*: If two materials cross-react in their respective assays, then separate assays could be performed on a sample and the results of each corrected for the observed amount of the other (Llewelyn et al., 1977). This leads to a very cumbersome calculation, particularly if the standard curves are non-parallel and the method is unlikely to find a routine application.

(3) *Destruction of cross-reacting material*: For example, cross-reaction with testosterone is often a problem in assays for dihydrotestosterone (DHT). Permanganate oxidation can split the A-ring of testosterone to form a non-reactive di-glycol while DHT itself is unaffected (Jeffcoate, 1979). A similar, but rather complex approach, is the use of a second antiserum which binds only the cross-reacting substances (Pratt et al., 1979).

10.3. Non-specific non-specificity

This term refers to interference in an assay by factors other than those which can be clearly identified by their physicochemical similarity to the ligand. It may lead to an underestimate or, more commonly, an overestimate of the amount of endogenous ligand in a sample. Four basic mechanisms which can lead to non-specific non-specificity will be considered.

10.3.1. Presence of materials which interfere with the binder–ligand reaction

A variety of materials can interfere non-specifically with binder–ligand reactions. Examples include the presence of large amounts of highly charged molecules such as heparin; high concentrations of low M_r materials such as salt and urea; conditions of acid or alkaline pH; and presence of fatty acids. An example of such an effect is shown in Fig. 7.1.

10.3.2. Variations of blank values in samples

The nature of the fluid used in the assay can have a striking effect on the blank values. For example, with separation by organic precipitation the assay blank may be considerably higher in tubes containing whole serum than in those containing assay buffer; the values given by unknowns will then be lower than the true values (Fig. 10.6). Furthermore, the assay blank value may vary between different samples of the same fluid. This could be avoided by carrying out an assay blank determination on every sample (i.e., replicate tubes with sample and tracer but no antibody); this would be very tedious and in practice is usually unnecessary.

10.3.3. Destruction or sequestration of binder, tracer or ligand

In most systems the binder is relatively stable. However, at least three mechanisms can grossly affect the performance of the tracer: enzymic destruction; absorption to surfaces; and binding by endogenous binders. Enzymic destruction is an important factor in assays using iodinated proteins or small peptides. These are highly susceptible to hydrolysis by enzymes in normal plasma or serum, a process which leads to a reduction in binding

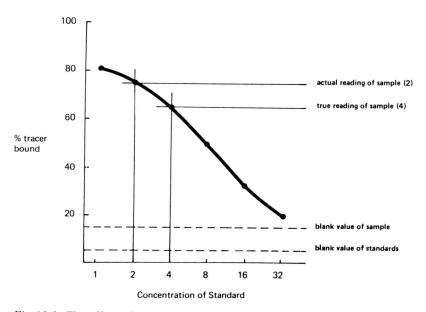

Fig. 10.6. The effect of a variable blank value on the specificity of a binding assay. If the blank value for the sample is higher than that of the standard, then the result obtained will be artefactually low. This problem is largely avoided if the composition of the standards and unknowns is identical.

which may be difficult to distinguish from that produced by unlabelled ligand (Fig. 10.7). Absorption to surfaces, such as those of glass tubes and syringes, is also common with small peptides and haptens, and the surface may 'compete' with the binder for tracer or unlabelled ligand and thus produce a variety of artefacts. Finally, biological samples may themselves contain binders — either the naturally occurring binding proteins (see § 7.5) or specific antibodies to the ligand (some insulin-treated diabetics) or the binder (7% of healthy subjects have circulating antibodies to sheep immunoglobulins; Hunter and Budd, 1980). These endogenous binders can lead to grossly discrepant results because of competition for the tracer.

The effects described above may also apply to the unlabelled ligand.

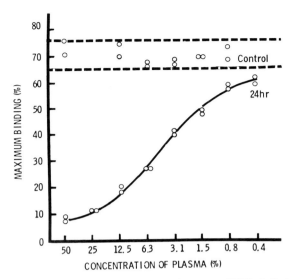

Fig. 10.7 The effect of enzyme destruction of a tracer. ^{125}I-Labelled oxytocin is incubated with an antiserum to oxytocin and varying concentrations of human late-pregnancy plasma (horizontal axis). After 24 h there is virtually no bound hormone in those tubes containing the highest concentrations of plasma. As the sample contained no oxytocin the loss of immunoreactivity is entirely due to destruction of the tracer by the placental enzyme, oxytocinase.

This applies particularly during the process of collection, preparation, and storage of the samples (see § 7.7).

10.3.4. The detection and elimination of non-specific non-specificity

The traditional method for detecting non-specificity of any type is the examination of parallelism between dilutions of sample (unknown) and standard. But, as with specific non-specificity, this should not be relied upon to guarantee identity.

The best approach to the elimination of non-specific non-specificity is to ensure that the composition of the standards is identical to that of the unknowns. If the fluid examined is serum and standards are prepared in ligand-free serum then problems are unlikely to occur. However, difficulties arise with fluids of variable composition, such as urine, or, more important, when a source of ligand-free fluid is not readily available. There are two potential sources of ligand-free fluid:

(1) The best is from a subject in whom none of the ligand is present: for instance, in the case of a drug, from an untreated patient; in the case of a hormone, from a subject in whom the gland of origin has been removed, or in whom production has been inhibited by an appropriate drug (e.g., dexamethasone suppression of ACTH); in the case of a placental product, from a non-pregnant subject.

(2) To use fluid from which endogenous ligand has been removed by absorption, such as the removal of insulin or thyroxine from serum by pre-treatment with charcoal. However, the absorption process may also remove non-specific interfering factors and the 'hormone-free' serum may not be strictly comparable to fresh normal serum.

If total comparability between sample and standard cannot be guaranteed, and in particular if a reliable source of ligand-free fluid is not available, there are a number of additional approaches to the elimination or at least the identification of non-specificity. Careful attention to assay technique can eliminate many potential sources of error. Factors such as absorption of tracer or unlabelled ligand to the surface of tubes can be identified by adding and removing tracer ligand from the tube, and estimating the proportion of counts which remain. It is usually possible, by trial and error, to select a tube which does not show this phenomenon. Enzymic destruction can be at least partly eliminated by the incorporation in the incubation mixture of enzyme inhibitors such as Trasylol. Extraction and concentration of ligand, (Ch. 7) can transfer material from an ill-defined environment such as urine or a tissue extract into a well-defined aqueous buffer system. As already noted, however, extraction itself may yield non-specific effects.

One of the traditional ways to eliminate non-specific non-specificity is to dilute the sample. Indeed, it is frequently taken as a rule-of-thumb that the sample should never constitute more than 10—20% of the total incubation volume. However, the greater the sample dilution, the poorer is the sensitivity, and it has been suggested by Hunter and Bennie (1979) that the best approach is to *increase* the amount of sample. This certainly applies if, as is frequently the case, the non-specificity or 'noise' yields a response curve less steep than the standard. Under these circumstances,

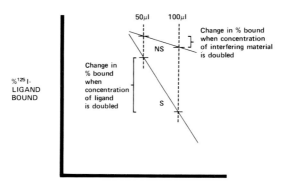

CONCENTRATION OF STANDARD (log scale)

Fig. 10.8. Why *increasing* the sample volume may decrease the non-specific non-specificity in an assay. The diagram shows the response curve for authentic ligand (S) and the non-parallel and less steep response curve for the interfering material (NS). It also shows the expected responses for sample volumes of 50 μl and 100 μl. Note that the change in % bound for the ligand with increasing sample concentration is much greater than that of the interfering material, and that the latter will therefore make less relative contribution at the highest sample concentration.

the greater the sensitivity the less will be the relative contribution of the noise (Fig. 10.8).

Physicochemical studies may also be of value to determine the precise nature of material measured in an assay. For example, the demonstration that the material inhibiting the binder—ligand reaction has the same properties as the authentic material in several systems of chromatography can greatly enhance the confidence in any results obtained (Fig. 10.9). Finally, and perhaps most importantly, it is critical with any system to examine the biological specificity of the results. In other words, that the answers obtained with the assay are comparable to those which would be expected from other information on the ligand in question. For example, it is possible with many hormones to obtain an indirect estimate of their circulating levels from a knowledge of the half-life in the circulation and the amount of administered exogenous material which will produce maximal end-organ response. If the apparent levels measured in an assay are greatly in excess of indirect estimates then it is likely that non-specific

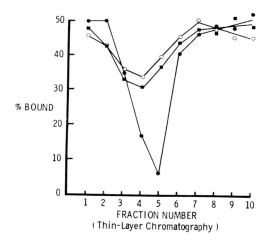

Fig. 10.9. Thin-layer chromatography of an extract of urine after adsorption to and elution from glass beads (see § 7.1.2 and Table 7.1). Each segment of the plate was extracted with 1 ml 60% (w/v) aqueous acetone. The extract was dried, dissolved in an aqueous buffer solution, and incubated with 0.05 ng ^{125}I-labelled oxytocin and a rabbit antiserum to oxytocin at a final concentration of 1 in 4,000. (o——o) Urine with no added hormone; (■——■) urine with added synthetic oxytocin; (●——●) synthetic oxytocin alone run on the same plate. Note that the elution patterns of endogenous material and recovered exogenous material are virtually identical. Neither, however, is identical to synthetic oxytocin alone, indicating some alteration of the material after addition and extraction from urine.

factors are operative. Similarly, the estimated levels should show appropriate variation under physiological or pathological conditions. For instance, material recorded as 'basal levels' of ACTH should be reduced or disappear following administration of corticosteroids.

CHAPTER 11

Characteristics of binding assays – precision

11.1. Definitions

The aim of a binding assay is to give the 'true' concentration of a ligand in a biological fluid. In practice, however, the actual result will diverge from the 'true' result because of imprecision on the one hand, and inaccuracy on the other. It is worthwhile to define these two terms because they are often confused (see also Fig. 11.1). 'Precision', also referred to as 'reproducibility', is a measure of the variation observed between repeated determinations on the same sample. 'Accuracy'*, is the degree to which the estimate approximates the true value: this is related to the specificity of the assay. Thus, an assay in which the endogenous ligand reacts differently from the standard and tracer ligands will always (unless correction factors are incorporated) be inaccurate however precise it may be. Accuracy can therefore be thought of in broadly the same terms as specificity (Ch. 10). This section will be concerned primarily with precision – the factors affecting precision, and the means for assessment and improvement.

---

* There is some confusion over the definition of the word 'accuracy'. Many workers, and the International Federation of Clinical Chemistry (Buttner et al., 1975) use the term as it is described here. Others, however, prefer to use the word 'bias' to describe the approximation to a true value, and 'accuracy' as a rather nebulous term which includes both bias and precision according to the equation:

$$\text{Accuracy} = \sqrt{\text{Bias}^2 + \text{Precision}^2} \tag{1}$$

This author prefers the first definition.

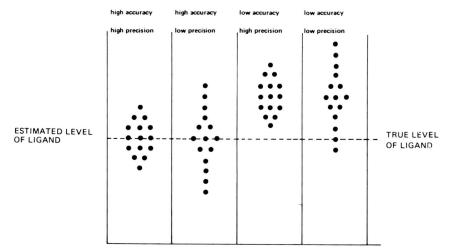

Fig. 11.1. The concepts of precision, variability of repeated determinations and accuracy (degree to which a measured concentration corresponds to the true concentration of a substance).

11.2. Factors affecting precision

These can be considered under two headings: errors due to the nature of the reagents and assay design; and errors arising in the actual operation of the assay. In practice, of course, the two are very closely related.

11.2.1. Errors in the reagents and design of the assay

11.2.1.1. Errors in the reagent solutions Imprecision due to a fault in the reagent solutions themselves is very rare. For this reason the common practice of comparing the precision of different assays on the basis of the difference between replicates is largely irrelevant. The major factor affecting this difference is the technical skill of the operator (or machine) which is unrelated to the reagents themselves. However, a specific error which can, but should not, arise is inadequate mixing of the primary reagents; this can lead to heterogeneity of the solution and of aliquots subsequently dispensed from this solution. Heterogeneity of this type is often seen when frozen material is thawed, or when lyophilised material is redissolved.

11.2.1.2. Errors due to the separation procedure The separation procedure can have a considerable effect on the precision of an assay. Certain types, notably the coated tube methods (§ 6.3.6.1), can sometimes give severe problems of reproducibility. Less well recognised is the influence of the assay blank value on precision, an effect which will apply with any separation technique. The assay blank value, as all other parameters, shows variation: some of this is due to technical errors, but an important part is due to variation between different unknown samples. Let us assume that the variation attributable to this factor is equivalent to 10% of the counts in the blank tubes. This will have almost no effect on the precision of an assay with an assay blank of 1% (variation 0.1%) and a zero standard of 50%. However, it will have a very substantial effect on an assay with a blank of 15% (variation 1.5%) and a zero standard of 30%. For this reason separation procedures characterised by high blank values (chiefly the chemical precipitations of the bound fraction such as ethanol, ammonium sulphate) should not be used in assays with a low '0' standard value (less than 40% of total counts).

The basic design of a separation procedure can also have an important influence on precision. This should be so arranged that the exact amount of the separating agent is not critical: for example, with an organic solvent added in a nominal volume of 1 ml, the addition of 0.8 ml or 1.2 ml should make little or no difference to the results. If this volume is non-critical over a reasonably wide range, one potential source of error is eliminated (Fig. 11.2).

11.2.1.3. Errors due to disequilibrium Most binding assays are incubated to equilibrium, but there are circumstances in which it may be desirable to separate bound and free ligand before equilibrium is achieved (§ 9.2.5). This is a potential source of imprecision: if the time taken for separation represents a substantial part of the total assay time, then the possibility arises of significant differences between the first and last tubes of an assay.

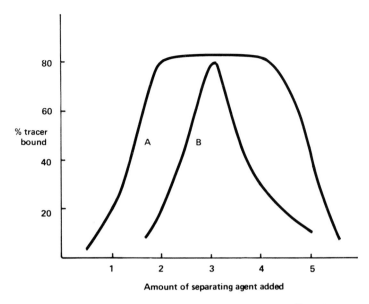

Fig. 11.2. Diagrammatic illustration of how precision can be affected by a separation procedure. With system B, small variations in the amount of separating agent added would have a substantial effect on the observed distribution of bound and free ligand. With system A, there is a long plateau where the amount of separating agent is non-critical, and even substantial errors would not affect the result. Systems of type A are much to be preferred.

11.2.1.4. Error due to standards The major error which can arise from the primary reagents is in the standards (see Das, 1980). The rules for and pitfalls in the preparation of standards have already been described (Ch. 2).

11.2.1.5. Errors at different points on the standard curve The precision of a binding assay varies according to the dose level measured, being at its best in the central part of the standard curve and declining at the extremes (Fig. 11.3). Assays should be designed so that the values of greatest clinical interest are measured with the greatest precision (see § 9.4).

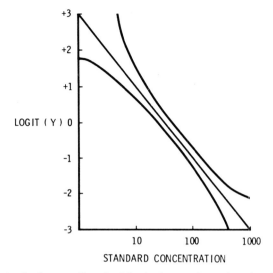

Fig. 11.3. A standard curve linearised by logit transformation showing the confidence limits to the curve. Note that these are much broader at the extremes and that precision is correspondingly reduced for these values.

A related question is whether or not the absolute precision varies at different parts of the standard curve — 'absolute precision' being defined here as the variation between replicates. There is, in fact, little evidence to suggest that it does, apart from that variation which can be attributed to the errors of different count rates.

11.2.1.6. Counting errors   Counting errors are an important source of imprecision in a binding assay using radioactive tracer. However, it is often assumed that they are the only source of variation when in fact the technical errors described in § 11.2.2 are considerably more important. Counting errors are of two types — those due to the equipment, and those intrinsic to the counting process itself. Errors attributable to the equipment are very rare: failures in up-to-date electronics, when they occur, are usually total and very obvious. Large fluctuations in the power supply may, however, give rise to problems. Equipment errors may also arise, particularly with well-crystals, if the volume of fluid counted varies widely; but in most assays a fixed volume of fluid or precipitate is examined, and counting geometry is therefore equivalent for all tubes. The intrinsic counting error is much the most important source of variation, and applies regardless of the nature and quality of the equipment. Radionuclide disintergrations are random events and therefore follow a Poisson distribution for which the standard deviation is equivalent to the square root of the total number of counts accumulated. In practical terms this implies that if repeated counts are performed on the same radioactive sample, then 95% (i.e., ± 2 standard deviations) of the values will lie within the mean ± the square root of the mean. Thus the error of any given number of counts can be calculated directly without recourse to experiment.

The implications of this for a selection of different total counts are shown in Table 11.1. The gain is precision between 10,000–100,000 counts is small, and that between 2,000–10,000 counts is not large relative to other errors in the assay. Furthermore, the counting error is independent of other errors and not a simple addition to them. For example, if technical errors are responsible for a 2% variation, and the number of counts accumulated is 10,000, then total error is only 2.2%; for 2,000 counts it is 3%. On this basis the precision of most assays will be perfectly satisfactory if the range of counts over the standard curve lies between 2,000–10,000. Only rarely will a system be of such basic technical excellence that anything is gained by the accumulation of larger

TABLE 11.1

The theoretical counting error for different numbers of total counts; the error is the square root of the total counts expressed as a percentage of the total counts

Total counts	Error (%)
100,000	0.3
50,000	0.4
20,000	0.7
10,000	1
5,000	1.4
2,000	2.2
1,000	3.2
500	4.5

totals. Long counting times and high numbers of counts are no substitute for correct performance of other steps of an assay. Counters should be regularly examined to ensure efficient operation. With single-well sample changers background readings should be taken in every sample position to identify contamination. With multi-head counters, the same tube should be counted repeatedly in each well to identify differences in detector efficiency.

11.2.2. Errors in the technical operation of the assay

For a well-designed system using adequate reagents, technical errors are much the most important course of variation.

Technical errors can be divided into major and minor. Major errors include failure to add reagent or sample to a tube, misidentification of samples, or serious faults in the calculation of results. Such errors are usually, but not necessarily always, recognised by the operator. The relevant samples or complete assay is repeated and the results are usually excluded from any calculation of 'between-assay' variation.

More important, because they are less easily identified or corrected, are the minor errors which occur because of the inevitable variability in the repetitive sampling and dispensing operations of which a binding assay consists. The errors arise both in the equipment used and in the operator using it.

(1) *Equipment errors:* Two main types of equipment are currently used for repetitive sampling and dispensing: the hand-held sampler/dispenser with a piston and spring return, and the motor-driven syringe (see Appendix I). If well maintained and operated correctly, the best models of these are reproducible to within 0.5% or better; indeed, it is often difficult to measure the error because it is equivalent to or less than that of the eventual system of detection (e.g., an analytical balance). However, the excellence of the equipment should be regularly examined and not simply assumed. This is especially important with older equipment to assess wear and tear. Accuracy is tested by dispensing a fixed volume of deionised water and weighing this on an analytical balance. Precision is tested by dispensing 20 aliquots of a fixed volume of radioactive tracer, counting each aliquot, and calculating the coefficient of variation of these counts. The figure obtained should be corrected for the intrinsic counting

error, which is equivalent to the square root of the mean counts for all aliquots. Variation should be 1% or better. Maintenance and cleaning is also essential — traces of dirt around plungers and pistons can lead to discontinuity of action and serious dispensing errors.

(2) *Operator errors*: The vast majority of minor errors in a radioimmunoassay can be firmly and exclusively attributed to the operator. Two well-known facts make this quite clear:

(*i*) There is often a notable difference in the precision obtained by two or more operators using the same reagents on the same day. The difference is at least partly related to experience: the novice can rarely equal the expert.

(*ii*) Precision will usually decline as increasing numbers of tubes are set up — a fatigue factor. As a rule of thumb, the maximum number of tubes set up manually in a day should not exceed 500 per operator.

The exact nature of the errors involved are usually difficult to identify but may include failure of adequate mixing, leaving drops of reagent on the sides of the tube or the tip of a pipette, and variability in the decanting or aspiration of supernatants. It is for these reasons that operator error can apply equally to the use of both hand pipettes and manually operated motor-driven pumps.

11.3. Quality control to monitor the precision of a binding assay

Quality control has been defined as 'the analytical and other steps which must be taken to ensure that results are of maximum clinical value' (Challand et al., 1974). Commonly used quality control parameters are shown in Table 11.2. Instrument statistics have already been considered.

11.3.1. Result statistics

Precision has already been defined as 'a measure of the variation observed between repeated determinations on the same sample'. This is an operative definition of the most important procedure used: repeated measurements on a quality-control pool. The results are often referred to as 'between-assay' or 'inter-assay' variation.

TABLE 11.2
Quality-control parameters commonly used in radioimmunoassays
(from a classification suggested by G.S. Challand)

Internal quality control:
1. Result statistics (quality-control samples, assay 'means', intuition) (§ 11.3.1);
2. Standard curve statistics ('0' standard, assay blank, mid-point, slope) (§ 11.3.2);
3. Replicate statistics (difference between replicates, quality-control samples) (§ 11.3.3);
4. Instrument statistics (counting errors) (§ 11.2.1.6 and 11.2.2).

External quality control (§ 11.5)

The single most important parameter, for internal or external schemes, is the result of repeated determinations on a quality-control pool.

11.3.1.1. Preparation of quality-control materials The sample or samples used for monitoring precision should have the following characteristics.

(1) They should consist of pooled samples containing endogenous ligand in the biological fluid for which the assay is intended (e.g., serum). Samples which are made up by addition of purified ligand to ligand-free fluid or diluent are not strictly speaking quality controls — rather they are standards; nevertheless, the vast majority of commercially available controls are of this type.

(2) The pooled samples should be available in substantial quantities, and should be aliquoted in such a way that the same basic pool will suffice for many months or even years of operation.

(3) The pooled samples should be stored at the lowest available temperature. Lyophilisation is not wholly desirable for the reasons given in Ch. 2, though it has immense practical advantages. Stability is difficult to prove: to determine whether a substance is stable under given conditions for a period of years requires an experiment lasting several years, and a reference system which is definitely stable. The latter purpose is served by the use, where available of 'biological pools' (see (5) below).

(4) Optimally, the pools should be chosen in such a way that their concentration represents high, medium and low values in the assay. This

provides an on-going check of precision at different parts of the standard curve (see Fig. 11.3 and 11.6).

(5) If possible, samples for quality-control pools should be collected from subjects under defined conditions: for example, a pool for plasma oestriol could be derived from normal subjects at the 36–40th weeks of pregnancy. The great advantage of this 'biological pool' is that it can always be repeated. Materials may alter with prolonged storage; physiology does not change. But there are many situations in which 'biological pools' are not readily available – for instance, in an assay for the blood levels of a drug. Under these circumstances quality-control pools can be prepared from assayed samples. If the range of ligand concentrations measured is 20–80 (taking quite arbitrary units), then 3 appropriate pools can be made from the residue of samples reading 20–40, 40–60 and 60–80. The problem with such pools is that the mean value may not easily be reproducible on another occasion.

(6) All the concepts presented here can be equally applied to the preparation of quality-control pools for use in several laboratories, or as part of national or supranational quality-control schemes or commercial schemes (Appendix II).

11.3.1.2. Analysis of result statistics   Between-assay variation is based on estimations of aliquots from the quality-control pool in every assay run. For this purpose the pool is treated as a single sample, i.e., if samples are assayed in duplicate, the control should also be examined in two tubes. The practice of running larger numbers of replicates of the control will give a falsely optimistic impression of precision; in large assays involving large numbers of tubes the control samples can be reintroduced at regular intervals to monitor drift. As a rule of thumb, one set of quality control samples should be included with every 30 patient samples. If the number of patient samples exceeds 100, it is a good practice to repeat the standard curve in a later part of the assay.

When a series of observations has been accumulated in successive assays there are a number of ways in which the results can be presented.

(1) *As a coefficient of variation (mean/standard deviation × 100):*   For most systems this will lie between 8–20%, assuming that the figure ap-

plies to a long series of assays, performed by different operators, and allowing for several batch changes in all the primary reagents (antibody, tracer, standards, and separation system). Lower estimates are frequently given, but will almost invariably be found to refer to a study limited on a single batch of reagents and one operator: the real practical value of this estimate must take into account such changes. Between-laboratory variation, assessed in the same manner, will almost invariably exceed 20%.

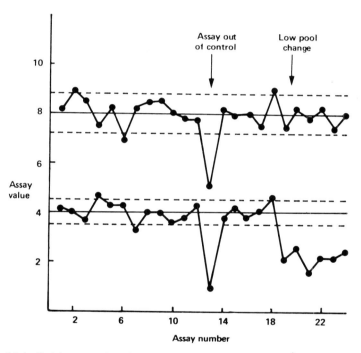

Fig. 11.4. Serial assay values for high-level and low-level quality control pools in a routine assay for hPL. The means and confidence limits to these values are shown. With a poorly executed assay both pools gave results well below the cumulative range; this assay was rejected. After replacement of the low level pool the values for this pool showed a marked decrease. However, because the results of the high level pool remained stable it was assumed that this change represented a true shift and was not due to poor control of the assay.

(2) *As a graph showing the serial values (Fig. 11.4)*: This is of great value in the individual laboratory since it is simple to plot and easy to comprehend. The value is further enhanced if the limits of the control pool, expressed as the mean and coefficient of variation, are also included. It should be placed in a prominent position where it can be easily seen by all concerned with the assay. It serves to indicate not only when a given assay run is out of control but also, if one pool is changed, whether or not an observed shift is affecting the assay as a whole.

(3) *As a cusum plot (Fig. 11.5)*: The 'cusum' is the cumulative sum of the differences of serial values from the progressive mean of that series.

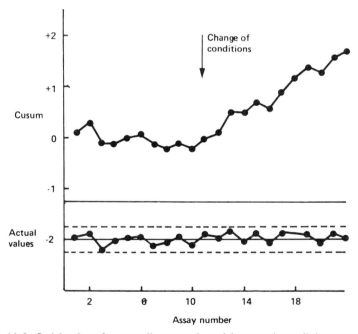

Fig. 11.5. Serial values for a quality-control pool in a routine radioimmunoassay for hPL (below) and the 'cusum' of these values (cumulative sum of the difference from the mean) (above). Note that the cusum plot is a much more sensitive indicator of a change in conditions than is the plot of serial values.

This is rather more difficult to construct than the simple graph of serial results, but is in many ways more instructive since it reveals very clearly a systematic but minor deviation in the assay.

(4) *Assay means*:   The mean of all results in a given assay can be used as a quality control parameter. It assumes that on any one occasion the composition of the samples examined will be similar, i.e., will contain similar numbers of high, normal and low results. This will usually apply only if there are relatively large numbers in the assay run; with small numbers (50 or less) the parameter is likely to be unstable and therefore unsuitable as a quality control. An alternative is the use of a 'restricted population mean' – samples for the assay are chosen on the basis of criteria which will yield a homogeneous population. In practice this is likely to be time-consuming and demands patient information which is often not available to the laboratory.

(5) *Intuition*:   This is an extension of the above approach, but in particular that of examining the assay mean and distribution. For example, an alert technologist notices an unusual preponderance of samples with abnormal results, i.e., in the 'hyper' or 'hypo' range and decides to repeat the assay. As a means of quality control this would be deprecated by the more mathematically inclined assayist. However, for those laboratories whose technologists are not intimately familiar with the comparison of frequency distributions by the Kolmogorov-Smirnov test, an intuitive approach may have some merits.

It should be strongly emphasised that the use of 'quality' control charts of any type does not evaluate the true 'quality' of an assay, but only its stability. 'Quality', in the sense of giving the best possible answers for clinical use, can only be achieved by careful attention to optimisation of reagents and protocol at the time the assay is first established.

11.3.2. Standard curve statistics

(1) *Blank values*:   The zero standard and assay blank should always be noted and if they fall outside limits set by previous experience then the fault must be identified before further runs are performed. A common cause of deviation is the use of outdated tracer which in all systems leads

to a fall in the zero standard, and in some to a simultaneous increase in the assay blank.

(2) *Intercepts on the standard curve*: The commonest example of this is the mid-point – the standard dose at which (percentage bound/percentage bound in '0' standard) is equal to 0.5 (ED_{50}).

(3) *Slope of the standard curve*: This can only be usefully estimated if the curve is linearised (e.g., by the logit transformation, see § 8.3). The information it gives is rather similar to that of the blank values, i.e., if the zero standard falls and/or the assay blank rises then the result is a decrease in slope.

(4) *The precision profile (or 'response–error relationship') (Ekins, 1978)*: Precision is estimated at various points on the standard curve by examining large numbers of replicates at these points. The results are plotted as a 'precision profile' (Fig. 11.6). This is a useful approach at the stage of initial assay design since it permits a choice of conditions which will minimise errors at dose levels which are considered to be particularly critical for clinical diagnosis.

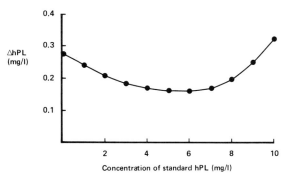

Fig. 11.6. A 'precision profile' for an hPL assay. Replicate determinations for 11 dose levels from 0–10 mg/l yield the errors (ΔhPL) shown on the vertical axis. This demonstrates that the best precision is obtained between 4–7 mg/l, with a progressive deterioration towards the extremes of the range.

11.3.3. Replicate statistics

(1) *Differences between replicates*: It is good practice to place an arbitrary upper limit on the difference between replicates, above which the result is ignored and the sample repeated. A typical figure for this limit would be 5% of the total counts in the system. The major purpose of this control is to eliminate figures one of which is probably grossly in error due to a fault in pipetting or counting. The fact that such faults occur not infrequently in both manual and semi-automatic assays is an excellent argument for the routine performance of replicates on every sample, standard and quality control.

(2) *Within-assay variation*: A series of determinations are made on a quality-control pool within the same assay, treating the pool identically with samples. Thus if the samples are normally estimated in duplicate a series of duplicate tubes are made up from the pool; the number of pool tubes should be at least 20 (i.e., equivalent to 10 samples in the same assay) and they should be spaced out between other samples in the assay to take account of the possibility of drift. The mean and standard deviation of all the estimates on the pool are calculated, and the result is expressed as a coefficient of variation (the standard deviation expressed as a percentage of the mean). For most systems this figure will be found to lie between 3–8%.

Within-assay variation can also be assessed as the coefficient of variation of duplicate samples:

$$\sqrt{\Sigma\left(\frac{d}{\bar{x}} \times 100\right)^2 / 2N}$$

where d = the difference between duplicate estimates

$\bar{x}$ = the mean of duplicate estimates

N = the number of duplicate estimates

This can be applied to any routine assay simply by analysing the results of samples falling within a certain dose range, e.g., levels which lie on the central part of the standard curve. It can be extended to all samples by including a factor which takes account of the slope of the standard curve at a given dose level (Rodbard, 1978) but this would require fairly extensive computational facilities.

The routine use of a test of within-assay precision can be strongly recommended because it may reveal that an assay is 'out of control' despite the fact that the mean values for quality control pools appear to be satisfactory (Wilson et al., 1979).

11.4. Practical use of a quality-control scheme

A quality-control scheme cannot be solely observational; sooner or later it will be necessary to take action based upon the results, i.e., to reject an assay which is 'out of control'. The question then arises, what are the criteria for taking such action?

The principle behind the establishment of such criteria can be illustrated by a simple example. A laboratory runs a routine assay in which it includes a quality control at a single dose level. When a number of assays have been performed the mean and standard deviations are calculated for the serial values. In subsequent work any assay for which the control result lies more than 2 standard deviations from the mean is rejected and repeated.

Unfortunately, the above example is a gross over-simplification of what can prove an extremely complex subject. The additional problems include:

(1) *A substantial number of assays have to be done before there is any firm basis for the analysis*: No action can be taken on the results of a quality control scheme until experience has accumulated. On the traditional rule that at least 30−50 figures are required for a meaningful calculation of variance, this would be the number of assays needed *before* control limits can be drawn.

(2) *The variation may not be normally distributed*:   Indeed, for immunoassay data it is more likely to be log-normal, and results should probably be analysed after logarithmic transformation or by a non-parametric approach using centiles.

(3) *The aim of rejection is to eliminate 'outliers'*:   Yet it is very difficult to distinguish between a true outlier and the extremes of a normal

distribution (see Healy, 1979). For example, in the simple case set out above, 1 in 20 assays would be rejected; these would certainly include the outliers, but in addition must include a proportion of assays which are statistically valid (i.e., they cannot be distinguished from all previous assays). Setting broader limits (e.g., 3 standard deviations) does not solve this problem, it merely reduces the number of rejected assays.

(4) *The example given does not help when there are several quality-control samples*: A typical routine assay may contain controls at 3 dose levels; what happens when one is outside limits and the remainder are satisfactory? There is no soundly based answer to this, but a typical rule-of-thumb might be to reject when two or more levels are outside control limits.

(5) *There are several other precision parameters, apart from serial estimates on quality-control pools*: Any of these may be outside limits and on its own would indicate rejection. The reductio ad absurdum is that if sufficient independent parameters are accumulated, then on statistical grounds at least one of them will be wrong in every assay. It is here that intuition must inevitably play a part, though commendable attempts are being made to systematise the subject [see 'Radioimmunoassay and Related Procedures in Medicine 1977' Vol. II, pp. 3–167, International Atomic Energy Agency, Vienna (1978)].

11.5. External quality-control schemes

The techniques of quality control described above were designed for internal use in individual laboratories. But with the massive growth in the clinical applications of radioimmunoassay there is an increasing number of 'external' schemes in which a designated centre, often government sponsored, is responsible for monitoring quality control in a number of laboratories. The basic methods of an 'external' scheme are very similar to those already described, viz. the distribution of aliquots from quality-control pools, and the on-going analysis of the data as it is returned. However, the type of information and its potential use may be quite different to that of an internal scheme.

(1) *Figures for within- and between-assay variation, based on coded samples without pre-assigned values, are invariably greater than those of internal schemes*:   This arises from the almost inevitable selection when quality-control samples are not examined 'blind'. Thus, an external quality-control scheme should be more truly representative of performance on individual patient samples received in the laboratory.

(2) *By evaluating the results from a number of different laboratories, it is possible to assess the 'bias' of results from any single laboratory*:   That is, the degree to which the results in an individual laboratory differ from the consensus of all participating groups. A strong positive or negative bias suggests that the performance of the laboratory is less than optimal. But this is not always the case: it is possible for a laboratory to have been among the first entrants to a new field and to have developed an un- rivalled experience and service based on absolute figures which, while analytically valid, differ substantially from that of later arrivals. Nevertheless, it must be accepted that consensus is highly desirable because:
(*i*) Bias is more usually due to poor performance than to unique expertise;
(*ii*) Clinical interpretation of results is much simpler and better if all laboratories produce similar values, and similar ranges for normal and abnormal.

(3) *An external scheme can provide positive critical feedback which is not available from an internal system (Fig. 11.7)*:   For example, a laboratory whose work is shown to be out of line with or notably poorer than that of other groups will be stimulated to improve its performance. In a good external scheme the central laboratory can often help with specific advice when this occurs.

(4) *An external scheme may reveal lack of consensus which can be attributed to the use of different reagents or different assay protocols*:   Under these circumstances it is reasonable to propose use of common reagents (standards, antiserum, tracer) and for a central laboratory to provide such reagents. Clearly this is more difficult to achieve in situations in which several manufacturers are competing for the supply of such reagents.

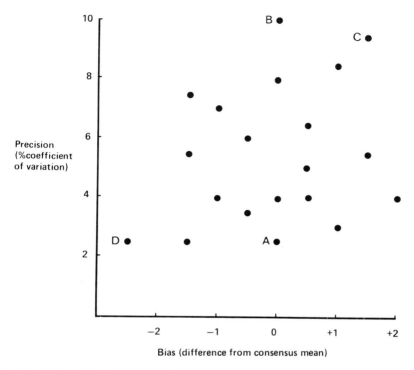

Fig. 11.7. A 'precision-bias' plot from an external quality scheme. Twenty laboratories make multiple replicate determinations on a single pool. The result from each laboratory is plotted as their observed variation (precision) versus the difference of their mean result from the group mean (bias). The interpretation of this can be illustrated by reference to the points identified as (A–D); laboratory (A), no bias and excellent precision; laboratory (B), no bias but poor precision; laboratory (C), a positive bias and poor precision; laboratory (D), negative bias but excellent precision.

A good example of an external scheme is that for human growth hormone provided by Dr W.M. Hunter under the auspices of the UK Supraregional Assay Service (Hunter and McKenzie, 1978). This has since yielded an improvement in between-laboratory precision from 40–30%. However, growth hormone represents a simple model because there is a well-established International Reference Preparation, a narrow range in normality and abnormality, no problem in obtaining antigen-free serum, and little or no variation between different batches of antiserum. For other analyses to which some of these problems do apply it is likely that the results of an external scheme would be little less than horrifying.

11.6. Summary – optimising the precision of a binding assay

The means for optimising the precision of a binding assay are very largely implicit in the factors which have already been described as affecting precision. However, it is worthwhile to re-emphasise certain points.

(1) The importance of monitoring precision by quality control – the principle feature of which should be the inclusion in every assay of aliquots from an appropriate pool. If there is no quality control, then there is no assay, because the operator has nɔ way of judging whether his results are of value or not.

(2) The importance of good assay design without which the best technician will obtain poor results regardless of the number and range of quality-control parameters.

(3) The importance of adequate training of the operator to ensure that simple technical errors are reduced to an absolute minimum. Automation, as discussed in Ch. 13, is some substitute for the operator, but will never be a complete substitute.

CHAPTER 12

Characteristics of binding assays – relation to other types of assay

12.1. Definitions

The perfect assay for a material in a biological fluid would consist of the extraction of the material at 100% purity and with 100% recovery, followed by weighing on a perfect balance. The result would be a true value of concentration as weight by volume which, if the M_r were also known, could be expressed as molar concentration.

No known assay even approaches this degree of perfection. In reality all assay work consists of a series of compromises and yields results which may approximate the true value but can never be guaranteed as so doing. In the final analysis the principle criterion is perhaps that of practicality – that the results should be useful in the biological or clinical context for which the assay is intended. This criterion serves to free the assayist from the concept that any one method is intrinsically superior to all others – for example, the inferiority complex which many radio-immunoassayists develop with respect to biological assay of hormones, when in fact the latter may deviate drastically from a real value because of the existence in a biological fluid of related but often unidentified materials.

The relationship between binding assays and other types of assay will be discussed according to the nature of the binder employed.

12.2. Receptor assays

Assays based on receptor binding proteins (see § 5.4) were introduced with much eclat because of their supposed close relationship to biological assay. However, certain reservations must be made about this relationship:

(1) Some receptors may apparently be different from those responsible for biological activity (Birnbaumer and Pohl, 1973);

(2) The receptor may be irrelevant to any known biological activity – an example is that which has been prepared from fat cells and which is capable of binding oxytocin;

(3) The possibility exists that a receptor might bind fragments of a molecule which are not biologically active – for instance, if part of the intact molecule binds to the receptor and function then depends on co-operative reactions with other parts of the intact molecule;

(4) The receptor may not bind a large pro-hormone molecule the measurement of which, in terms of physiology and pathophysiology, is likely to be just as important as the active molecule. For example, the radioreceptor assay for ACTH based on adrenal cortex receptors does not detect the ACTH-like material found by immunoassay in some patients with carcinomas not associated with an endocrine syndrome (Odell, 1978) and the sera of such patients contains high M_r material (22,000) which reacts in the ACTH immunoassay (Ratter et al., 1980);

(5) A receptor assay is unlikely to measure metabolites of an intact molecule – metabolites which, as in the case of the steroid conjugates, may be of considerable practical significance.

All these factors serve to emphasise that assays using cell receptors are not necessarily and intrinsically superior to assays based on other types of binder.

12.3. Assays using circulating binding proteins (CBP)

Naturally-occurring circulating binding proteins are quite distinct from receptors (see § 5.5). When used as a binding reagent they do not, therefore, reflect the biological activity of a molecule (though assays for circulating binders, using binding of ligand as the response parameter, are true biological assays). The results of CBP assays can show striking discrepancies from biological assays, a notable example being the measurement of folate derivatives using milk binding proteins (CBP assay) or Lactobacillus casei (microbiological assay) (Shane et al., 1980).

12.4. *Immunoassays for hormones*

The immense practical success of radioimmunoassays has led to the frequent criticism that they do not measure the functional activity of a molecule. Because the antibody-combining site is usually considerably smaller than the molecule to which the immunoassay is directed, only a small section of the molecule is actually measured, and this section may be remote from the part responsible for biological activity (Fig. 12.1). The possibility therefore arises that the immunoassay might measure inactive fragments and thereby overestimate the concentration of intact, active molecules. This phenomenon is usually referred to as the 'dissociation of immunological and biological activity'.

Several examples of this situation have been investigated in detail. Among the most familiar is adrenocorticotrophin (ACTH); the ACTH molecule contains 39 amino acids of which the first 24 are responsible for biological activity and are similar in all species, while the sequence 25–39 has no biological activity and differs between species. Antisera raised to the intact ACTH molecule are usually directed to a site in the inactive C-terminal portion of the molecule and will therefore potentially detect inactive fragments resulting from metabolic degradation of ACTH in vivo. In practice this problem is partly overcome by the use of antisera produced using synthetic 1–24 sequence (Synacthen, Ciba) as immunogen. With an antiserum of this type and a tracer of the same material, estimates of ACTH by radioimmunoassay are comparable to those of biological assay (Rees et al., 1973).

Another example is presented by the small peptide hormone oxytocin. The bulk of the molecule consists of a ring structure completed by

Functional site

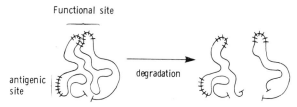

Fig. 12.1. Dissociation of immunological and biological activity. Splitting of the molecule has destroyed the functional site while leaving the antigenic site intact.

a disulphide bridge; biological activity depends on the ring structure though it is progressively destroyed by sequential removal of amino acids. When oxytocin is incubated in the presence of human late pregnancy plasma, which contains the enzyme oxytocinase, the rate of destruction as assessed by biological assay is greater than that by radioimmunoassay (James et al., 1971). A similar phenomenon is seen following an infusion of oxytocin in vivo, though here the major factor leading to destruction of the hormone is metabolism in the liver and kidneys (Fig. 12.2).

The degree to which dissociation of biological and immunological activity is likely will be highly variable according to the nature of the system studied. Where the antigenic site is coincident with the functional site little or no dissociation occurs. Where the sites are not coincident the amount of dissociation will depend on the relative rates of degradation of the two sites. If the functional site is less stable, then an immunoassay will over-estimate the total activity present. On the other hand, if the antigenic site is less stable the immunoassay will yield an underestimate – a situation which appears to be extremely rare in practice.

Dissociation of immunological and biological activity cannot always be explained on the basis of differences in the rate of degradation of the

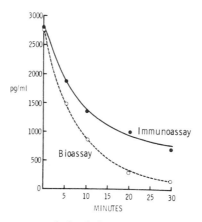

Fig. 12.2. The disappearance of circulating oxytocin, measured by immunoassay and bioassay, following an intravenous infusion of the hormone.

two sites concerned. An example which seems almost to defy analysis is that illustrated in Fig. 12.3; serial blood samples collected throughout the menstrual cycle and submitted to cytochemical bioassay and radioimmunoassay for luteinising hormone (LH) show a totally different pattern for the two types of measurement. Possible explanations include the existence of two forms of LH, or the presence at mid-cycle of factors which inhibit biological activity but do not affect immunological activity. Similar observations have been made with TSH; high levels of immunoreactive TSH have been observed without apparent bioactivity in some cases of hypothyroidism (Belchetz, 1976).

Though the dissociation of biological and immunological activity is often regarded as a disadvantage of the latter systems, it can also have possible advantages. In situations where biological material is highly unstable or has a very short half-life in vivo the specific measurement of its metabolic 'footprints' may be as valuable or more so than that of the

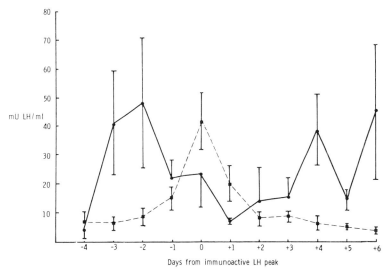

Fig. 12.3. Circulating levels of luteinising hormone (LH) in normal menstrual cycles as measured by immunoassay (■--- ■) and a cytochemical bioassay (●——●). Note the complete absence of any relationship between the two (from data kindly supplied by Dr. R.M. Kramer).

parent compound. A good example is the measurement of the prostaglandin metabolite 15-keto $PGF_{2\alpha}$ (Levine and Gutierrez-Cernosek, 1972). Another is the measurement of the biologically inert carboxy-terminal fragments of parathyroid hormone (PTH), which constitute more than 80% of the immunoreactive PTH in the plasma of patients with primary hyperparathyroidism; a clinically effective radioimmunoassay should be directed to these fragments (Benson et al., 1974; Di Bella et al., 1978).

12.5. Immunoassays for non-hormonal compounds

Though dissociation of biological and immunological activity is usually discussed in the context of hormones it may also apply to other materials. For example, enzymes are classically assayed by their biological 'activity' – the rate of conversion of a substrate to some easily measurable product; an example familiar to radioimmunoassayists is the estimation of plasma renin activity by the generation of angiotensin I. The factors contributing to this activity are often complex, depending not only on the precise conditions under which the determination is carried out, but also on the fact that several different enzymes may contribute to a given 'activity'. Immunoassays for enzymes have been described (e.g., for placental alkaline phosphatase – Jacoby and Bagshawe, 1972). Provided that the usual criteria of purity of antigen and specificity of the antiserum are met, these should measure the absolute concentration of a given enzyme independent of any of the factors which may influence its activity. The concept of 'enzymes by mass' is very attractive in practical clinical terms: for diagnostic as opposed to research purposes the functional activity is irrelevant except as a means to an end – which is to estimate the release of an enzyme into the blood as a result of cell damage (Landon et al., 1977). Immunoassay can do this directly. Furthermore, it raises the interesting possibility of distinguishing intracellular and circulating enzymes which have the same activity; specific measurement of the former in blood would be a much more sensitive indicator of trouble because it should not normally appear in this site (Fig. 12.4). Other examples of this approach are the measurement of circulating myoglobin or isoenzymes of creatine kinase in the diagnosis of myocardial infarction (Kagen et al., 1975; Roberts et al., 1977; Van Steirteghen et al., 1978; Zweig et al., 1978).

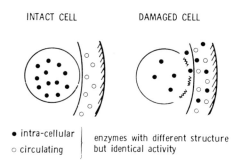

INTACT CELL   DAMAGED CELL

- intra-cellular   enzymes with different structure
○ circulating   but identical activity

Fig. 12.4. Why immunological activity may be of more practical value than biological activity. An enzyme exists in two forms, one intracellular and one extracellular. They have different chemical structures but identical functional activity. A classical assay could not distinguish these. However, an immunoassay which recognises structure and not function could specifically measure the intracellular enzyme and thus provide a very sensitive indicator for this enzyme when it appears in the circulation as a result of cell damage.

Since the antigenic site of an enzyme molecule may be quite separate from the active site there is, of course, no guarantee that an immunoassay will correlate directly with enzyme activity. However, assays specific to the active site have been described (e.g., urokallikrein, Silver et al., 1980) which show excellent correlation with function.

Many materials which are measured by radioimmunoassay have no biological activity in the sense in which this term is commonly used — examples include carcino-embryonic antigen, α-fetoprotein and the fibrin degradation products. Furthermore, for most compounds of this type there is no alternative system of assay for the concentration in biological fluids, and therefore no reference system against which to judge 'dissociation'. Under these circumstances, proof that the immunoassay is measuring the intended material and not some variant depends on physicochemical procedures of the type outlined in § 10.3.4 for the examination of specificity. The finding of non-identity does not necessarily invalidate the assay. For instance, the bulk of material measured in serum by an assay for the terminal degradation product of fibrin/fibrinogen, fragment E, is in fact material of higher M_r which represents partially degraded fibrinogen (Fig. 12.5). But since the use of fragment E has several technical advantages

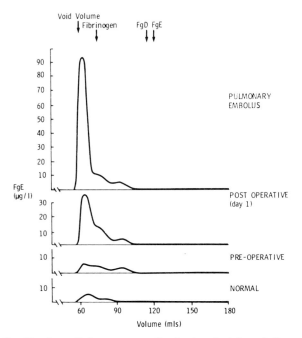

Fig. 12.5. Results of a radioimmunoassay for the terminal degradation product of fibrinogen, fragment E (FgE) when applied to fractions of human sera obtained by gel-filtration chromatography. Note that in both normal and abnormal cases the bulk of the endogenous material detected by this assay is of an M_r-value greater than that of fibrinogen itself, i.e. is not fragment E.

(availability and stability of reagents, specificity with respect to intact fibrinogen) the use of this system has many practical advantages.

With small molecules (haptens such as steroids and drugs) dissociation of biological and immunological activity is not a problem; the size of the molecule does not allow for any significant separation of the functional and antigenic sites. Thus, radioimmunoassays for antibiotics such as gentamicin and netilmicin (Broughton and Strong, 1976; Broughton et al., 1978) give results very similar to those of microbiological assays.

12.6. Conclusions

No assay is perfect, and different types of assay will reflect different aspects of the same material. Given that any assay should, during its development, be compared with other methods the final criterion must be — is it useful? There is little point in deprecating a technique because it yields results which are twice those of a more sophisticated procedure, when the former is simple and capable of high throughput. This has always been the great strength of radioimmunoassays over biological assays. Even if the result is not exactly 'right' according to some absolute reference, it is still immensely valuable if it serves to distinguish, on a routine basis, between health and disease.

CHAPTER 13

Automation of binding assays

13.1. Automation of binding assays

All binding assays consist of repetitive steps of reagent addition, mixing, separation, and counting of tubes. At the basic technical level this has been described as 'the scientific equivalent of sewing mailbags' (Bagshawe, 1975) and there can be no doubt that for the actual worker at the laboratory bench the performance of these assays is exceptionally tedious. But the disadvantages extend beyond a simple dislike of repetitive manual tasks:

(1) Endless repetition can very readily lead to loss of precision;

(2) Manual methods are labour-intensive and therefore expensive.

For these reasons a degree of automation or total automation of binding assays is highly desirable. The eventual aim should be that of any automated procedure in clinical chemistry — a sample, with appropriate identification, is put in at one end of a machine, and after the shortest possible lapse of time a result is printed out on a suitable form at the other end. The only demand on the routine operator should be the introduction of bulk reagent and general maintenance of the equipment (Table 13.1). It is also frequently the case that 'academic' innovators of automated technology suggest that their system will be simple and inexpensive because it can be built up from cheap, readily available components. Yet all past experience indicates that most customers, who are usually not mechanics, will demand a complete and ready-to-go package which in this area of technology is unlikely to cost less than $25,000, and might easily be 2−3-times this figure.

At present there is no widely used and fully accepted equipment for the performance of fully automated binding assays. However, this area is

TABLE 13.1

Characteristics of an ideal system for the automation of radioimmunoassay

---

1. Complete automation: The technologist introduces samples and reagents at the beginning, and no further action is required until the results are printed out at the end
2. Simplicity of operation
3. Reliability
4. Rapid sample throughput
5. Ability to handle large numbers of samples at a single loading
6. Flexibility to handle many different types of assay with a rapid changeover from one to the next
7. Flexibility to handle small numbers of samples (e.g., a single emergency estimation)
8. Economic use of reagents (minimal dead volumes)
9. Ability to use reagents from many different sources
10. Purchase price economic for an amortisation period of 5 years
11. Reasonable running costs (reagents and maintenance)

---

the subject of intensive development, not least in the activities of several large commercial organisations.

The general features of automated systems can best be described under the headings of the successive steps in a single binding assay: identification and dispensing of the sample; addition of reagents; incubation; separation of bound and free ligand; quantitation of the tracer; and calculation of results. The same headings also form the basis for discussion of the 'semi-automated' systems which are already in widespread use.

13.2. Identification and dispensing of the sample

There are two means for identification of patient samples in any assay: indirect by numbering of the samples and reaction tubes in a fixed sequence; and direct by labelling the reaction tubes with the information (patient's name and number) from the sample tube. Both types of procedure are used in manual assays, and both can be automated by the use of a digital computer. Identification by numerical sequence has the advantages of simplicity and convenience; the disadvantages are the possibility of serious mistakes due to an error in the sequencing, and that a list of all samples has to be compiled. In the case of a fully automated assay the list can be in the form of a punched tape prepared as the samples are introduced, and subsequently read out as part of the 'on-' or 'off-line' calculation of results. By contrast, direct labelling of the reaction tubes has the great advantage that it almost completely eliminates errors of identification. The disadvantage is that it requires, with a fully automated procedure, a very sophisticated system for labelling each reaction tube in machine-readable code; this is not available on any current equipment.

In most automated systems the sample is dispensed from tubes or cups set out in a tray – which may be in the form of a turntable or a rectangular cassette. Each position on the tray has a number which provides sample identification. A fixed amount of sample is aspirated from each tube of the reaction tray and transferred to the reaction tubes for mixing with reagents.

An important and serious difficulty of this step is that of carry-over from one sample to the next. A small residue of specimen in the delivery nozzle may be dispensed with the following specimen; if the first sample contains a high level of the substance being measured and the second a low level the contamination can seriously affect the results. This problem can be overcome to some extent by arranging that the delivery of a fixed volume of sample is followed by the delivery of a fixed and larger quantity of assay diluent through the same nozzle. In practice 'wash-ratios' of 3 : 1 or greater are required if significant carry-over is to be avoided between samples which differ in their concentration by an order of magnitude or greater.

Another problem at the step of sample dispensing is blocking of the aspiration tube with particulate material in the sample – especially when the latter is plasma. The operator working with a manual pipette can observe and correct this fault; a machine cannot and may dispense a sample volume which is considerably less than that intended.

13.3. Addition of reagents

The manner of addition of reagents will be determined by which of the two fundamental approaches to automation is adopted: a discrete system or a continuous-flow system. In a discrete system the sample and re-agents are delivered into an individual reaction tube (replicated if neces-sary) via a system of machine-driven syringes or roller pumps (i.e., a robot which reproduces manual movements). Current equipment of this type, which is fairly widely used as part of semi-automated systems, varies chiefly in whether the tubes are moved mechanically past a fixed delivery nozzle (as in the LKB 2071 and Micromedic systems) or whether the tubes remain static and the delivery nozzle is moved on a mechanical head; combinations are also possible (as in the Analmatic system). In continuous-flow systems (Technicon), the reaction mixture circulates in a length of tubing, successive samples or replicates being separated by a bubble. Flow is maintained by roller pumps, and reagents are introduced via side arms controlled by valves.

13.4. Incubation

This can be either 'off-line' or 'on-line'. For most current assays, in which incubation takes considerably longer than all other steps, an off-line approach is necessary. With discrete systems the reaction tubes are in a cassette which can be removed, stored under appropriate conditions, and then returned to the machine when incubation is complete. With a con-tinuous-flow system the flow can be stopped and the incubation coil removed and stored.

Automation, and particularly that of the continuous-flow type, is well suited to the type of 'disequilibrium' assay described in § 9.2.5. With careful design these can achieve exceptional sensitivity in very short in-cubation times, and the nature of a continuous-flow process is such that the reaction time for every sample is identical. Developments in this area are awaited with great interest.

13.5. Separation of bound and free ligand

This is one of the most time-consuming steps in a binding assay involving, as it almost invariably does, the addition of an agent to insolubilise bound or free ligand, centrifugation or filtration to separate the insoluble phase, and removal of the soluble phase prior to counting (see Ch. 6). It is the step which, more than any other, has proved difficult to automate, and current efforts in this direction can perhaps better be described as ingenious rather than perfect.

As there is no general approach to the automation of separation, the present available systems (reviewed by Ingrand, 1978) will be briefly summarised (see also Table 13.2).

(1) *Picker and Berchtold systems:* Following addition of the precipitating agent, the contents of the reaction tube are transferred to filter discs (cellulose acetate, polycarbonate, glass fibre, or paper) located on a flexible plastic tape supplied from a spool. The tape moves on to a station at which each filter is sealed on its lower surface to a vacuum chamber; the soluble phase is thus removed, leaving the insoluble phase

TABLE 13.2
Automated and semi-automated systems for radioimmunoassay

Name of system	Manufacturer
Semi-automated systems	
Analmatic	Searle (Baird and Tatlock)
Analmat	Gilson, France
Medicatome	CEA
Prias	Packard
Micromedic	Micromedic
UltraRIA	LKB
Centria	Union Carbide
'Southmead' system	—
Hydra RIA	Innotron
Automated systems	
Concept 4	Micromedic
Darias	Picker
RIA-E-600	Berchtold
Gammaflow	Squibb
STAR	Technicon
ARIA II	Becton Dickinson

on the filter which, after drying, is wound through a detector system for counting (Bagshawe, 1975; Marschner et al., 1975).

(2) *Centria system (Union Carbide)*: The contents of each reaction vessel are transferred to an individual pre-packed Sephadex column, the latter being mounted in groups in a centrifuge head. Centrifugation results in separation of the bound and free fractions by molecular-sieve chromatography (see § 6.3.2): the first fraction to emerge from the column (antibody-bound ligand) is then transferred for counting. Alternatively, the column consists of a solid-phase second antibody and the free fraction emerges (Meriadec et al., 1979).

(3) *Technicon 'STAR' system*: Based on the continuous-flow principle (see above), and on the use of antibody covalently linked to cellulose coated onto iron particles (Forrest, 1977). After incubation, the iron particles are held static by a magnetic field while the free phase is removed by washing. The particles are then released from the electromagnet and transferred (again by continuous-flow) to a counting head.

(4) *Technicon 'PACIA' system*: Determines agglutination of coated particles by light scattering (see § 4.1).

(5) *ARIA II system (Becton–Dickinson)*: Employs a reusable chamber containing solid-phase antibody. The sample and other reagents pass through this in a continuous-flow system, and the same chamber can be used for up to 3,000 tubes.

(6) *Gammaflow system (Squibb) (Brooker et al., 1976; Valdes et al., 1979)*: Employs a column containing an anion-exchange resin, with or without added charcoal, which adsorbs free antigen. The sample and other reagents pass through this in a continuous-flow system.

(7) *Micromedic systems 'Concept 4 Automatic Radioassay'*: Employs antibody-coated tubes (Johnson et al., 1976).

(8) *'Southmead system' (Ismail et al., 1978)*: This uses antibody covalently linked to porous agarose particles (size 40–70 μm). After mixing

and incubation, separation is achieved using a highly porous membrane (pore size 10 μm) mounted in a specially designed block. A precise amount of the filtrate (i.e., the free fraction) is quantitated in a γ-counter.

13.6. Counting of radioactivity

This does not differ in principle from the general methods described in Ch. 3. In the Picker machine the paper spool is wound between opposed pairs of crystal detectors; a total of 5 heads is available permitting the simultaneous counting of 5 locations on the tape. In the Centria system, 3 classical detector heads count 3 tubes at a time. In the Technicon machine, the tubing of the continuous-flow system is formed as a coil in a well-type crystal; each segment of magnetic particles is counted as it passed through this coil. In the Southmead system, the counter is triggered by the inclusion of a dye in the wash solution which is detected by a colorimeter interfaced to the counting head.

13.7. Calculation of results

Most currently developed or developing systems of automated RIA have full on-line computational facilities of the type described in § 8.6. The use of a fairly sophisticated computer is justified in this context because it can also undertake other functions including sequence timing in the machine itself and replacement of electronic components in the detector system.

13.8. Batch processing

A valid and highly attractive alternative to the automated systems described above is the use of semi-automated batch-processing systems. The principle of these is an extension of the 'multi-head' concept already described for γ-counters (see § 3.3). If all steps of an assay were carried out in a single modular rack (i.e., dispensing of sample and reagents, separation of bound and free ligand, and counting) then the rate of throughput would have a potential of many hundreds or even thousands of samples per hour. Ergonomically, the only additional work would be manual transfer of racks from one unit to the next, and even for a very large assay or series of assays this would involve no more than a few minutes of actual operator time. When it is also appreciated that such systems can be genuinely inexpensive it seems quite likely that the future of automated radioimmunoassay must reside with batch-processing systems.

13.9. Conclusions

Fully automated systems for binding assays are not at present widely available and, of the machines under development, it is difficult to predict which will become the 'market leader'. That such machines will be extensively used is, however, guaranteed by the exponential growth in the practical application of radioimmunoassays.

The principle advantages of automation are:

(1) High sample throughput (20–60/h) for a minimum of operator time – implicit in which is a reduction of costs because machines are usually less expensive than people;
(2) Increased speed of sample throughput – work does not need to be deferred, and the possibility exists of using fast disequilibrium assays;
(3) Increased precision through elimination of operator variation (see § 11.2.2).

The disadvantages are:

(1) Unless the machine is fully used the cost benefits are negated – for example, none of the equipment described above would be cost-effective in a laboratory receiving less than 50–100 samples/day;
(2) Several of the current systems are 'reagent dedicated', i.e., can only be used with the manufacturer's own kits because of the specialised nature of the separation process. For many buyers this will virtually eliminate any flexibility in the choice of reagents, and may commit them to unacceptably high running costs;

(3) If the machine breaks down (which it inevitably will from time to time) then the laboratory without sufficient technicians to process urgent samples manually will be in serious difficulties.

All these points should be examined with care before a decision, which will often be influenced by the current passion for hardware, is made.

Finally, it is not unlikely that batch processing systems will soon become the method of choice.

CHAPTER 14

Organisation of assay services

Most binding assays have long passed the stage of research procedures. There are now several branches of clinical medicine which could not be actively pursued without these techniques. Thus an important consideration is how to deliver the best possible service to the patient at the lowest possible price. The subject of this last chapter is the organisation of assay services. Although the discussion centres around radioimmunoassay similar observations would apply to non-isotopic techniques.

14.1. Who should perform radioimmunoassay?

The practice of medicine and pathology is highly structured on a departmental basis and when a new subject emerges there may be a period of years or even decades before it is formally recognised. Until a new subject comes of age, it will be practised under the aegis of an existing department and the final establishment of a new speciality can be a painful process at the personal and administrative levels. The breadth of application of radioimmunoassay has led to its emergence from departments as disparate as endocrinology, obstetrics/gynaecology, clinical chemistry, nuclear medicine, anatomy and physiology, and it is difficult to predict within any one hospital where one will find the radioimmunoassay laboratory; sometimes there are several. This may be satisfactory, indeed inevitable, at the research level. It is highly unsatisfactory when the demand is for a routine service to patients. The only place for routine radioimmunoassays is in a radioimmunoassay laboratory managed and staffed by people who are experts in radioimmunoassay. Whether this laboratory operates under the auspices of a department of clinical chemistry, or of nuclear medicine, or any other is immaterial – no existing department has any prior claim in the absence of experienced personnel.

Radioimmunoassay is a sufficiently large subject and sufficiently different from any other to merit full-time staff who are dedicated to this subject alone. A busy centre should have full-time personnel at all levels who are not expected to have a substantial and simultaneous commitment to routine clinical chemistry, to in vivo isotopic methods, or to a clinical discipline. Exceptions must, of course, be made for those situations in which the result is always required urgently — such as measurement of drug levels.

14.2. Organisation of an assay laboratory

Certain generalisations can be made on the requirements of a new laboratory:

(1) *Staff*:   The number of staff is determined by the throughput of assays. As a rule of thumb, one technician can process 5000 samples/year, or 100–150/working week. There are, of course exceptions: for assays with extraction steps, the throughput will be much reduced; for automated assays, it may be substantially greater. Similarly, the output of a technician who is responsible for several different types of assay will be less than that of one responsible for only a single assay. For every 3–4 technicians actively engaged in RIA procedures, the unit will require one well-trained graduate. Any size of unit will also require a full or part-time director who may be a medical or non-medical graduate with an extensive background in radioimmunoassay. At least one medical graduate should be involved in the interpretation of results.

There are many situations in which a laboratory will be required to perform radioimmunoassay procedures at throughputs considerably less than those suggested above (i.e., fewer than 250 samples/week). Examples would include the smaller district laboratory responsible for a small number of urgent determinations such as those required in the assessment of drug levels or for fetoplacental dysfunction. In these circumstances 2 or 3 members of the general laboratory staff should be deputed to become familiar with the use of reagent kits (see below), so that any one of them is able to meet demand on an ad hoc basis.

(2) *Staff training*: It is difficult to lay down any specific course of training for those involved in the management of a RIA laboratory other than that they should have a period of not less than one year in a recognised and active unit carrying out this type of work. Formal training schemes cannot substitute for experience, and the typical educational course now available can only provide a theoretical background to what is essentially a practical subject. Similarly, it is impossible to be specific about the type of person who should be trained – a graduate in almost any scientific discipline would be appropriate, with perhaps a slight edge towards the biochemist.

At the technical level the training problem is simpler. Any reasonably intelligent person with a secondary education in science subjects is suitable and can be introduced immediately to RIA techniques. No amount of previous experience and training in non-RIA subjects (e.g., medical physics, clinical chemistry) will qualify them any better. A young man or woman taken direct from school to work in a busy unit should be capable of independent running of an assay within 3 months and of several assays, if necessary, within a year. If well supervised and provided with a reasonable background of principle and practice, such people will be as competent and effective – often more so – than those with a long list of irrelevant qualifications.

(3) *Space*: The space requirements for a RIA laboratory do not differ significantly from those of any general analytical laboratory. A provision of 3–5 m of bench should be made for each person involved in the day-to-day handling of specimens together with additional areas for counters, centrifuges, automated equipment, sample reception and offices. A substantial unit with 12 staff and an annual throughput of 30,000–50,000 samples would be well-housed in a total area of 300 m^2*. A specific requirement of the larger unit (i.e., those performing their own iodinations) is a completely separate area reserved exclusively for the handling of high levels of radioactivity; the design of this area should conform to national and international regulations (see Appendix V).

---

* In developing countries particular attention may have to be given to the provision of a power-supply with stable voltage, and of air-conditioning

(4) *Equipment*: The specific requirements of a RIA laboratory are set out in Table 14.1.

(5) *Reagents*: The source of reagents will vary greatly with the size and type of laboratory. At one extreme is the very large group who prepare the majority of their own reagents and, may, indeed, distribute these to other laboratories. At the other extreme is the small group who use only 'kits' of reagents from outside suppliers. Between the two every possible combination of local and outside supply is encountered.

For laboratories performing RIA a key point is whether or not they have facilities for radioiodination. In the absence of these the unit is likely to be a predominantly kit user since there are few prime suppliers, either in the public or private sector, who are prepared to deliver tracer on its own. By contrast, the other reagents for RIA can be prepared relatively easily from stable bulk materials.

Many laboratories like to prepare their own reagents. This has two serious disadvantages:

(1) It has been repeatedly emphasised that no two sets of reagents, however apparently identical, will ever give exactly the same result. Discrepancy can be minimised and the value of the tests correspondingly enhanced if common sets of reagents and a common methodology are distributed from a central source.

TABLE 14.1
Principal items of equipment used in a radioassay laboratory

General laboratory items (e.g., balances) are not included

Single-well manual γ-counter
Multiple-well manual γ-counter *or* automatic sample changer
Centrifuge with temperature control and multi-tube capacity
Radiation monitor
Programmable calculator or microcomputer
Set of repeating micropipettes
Deep-freeze ($-20°C$) and refrigerator
Miscellaneous; air compressor, vortex mixer, magnetic stirrer, water bath, sample tubes, tube racks, laboratory glass and plastic ware

(2) It is often overlooked that the preparation of primary reagents is time-consuming and expensive. Oversimplified costings often ignore the major costs – labour and general overheads. As a rule of thumb, a throughput of less than 50 samples/week for a given assay does not merit local preparation of reagents – a kit will be more cost-effective and probably give better results.

Kits may be prepared either by public organisations or private firms – usually the latter. Commercial kits are often disparaged because of the high profit margins involved. This is an historic concept: over the last few years prices have not proved sensitive to inflation and margins are now comparable to those on most high-grade chemical reagents. However, the increasing and highly desirable control over the quality of kits by Government bodies will inevitably, as it already has with drugs, curb competition and thus lead to an increase in prices in real terms.

14.3. Organisation of assay services

The primary criteria for routine assay services are availability, efficiency, and cost, the three factors being closely related. Availability implies that an assay of clinical value, however recondite, should nevertheless be accessible to every clinician. Efficiency implies that the result should be available in the shortest possible time, and should have accuracy and precision such that it confers maximum clinical benefit. Finally, the cost should be as low as is compatible with the maintenance of an effective service.

In the first edition of this book proposals were made for a Government-sponsored scheme involving three 'tiers' of laboratories: supra regional, regional, and local. It is now apparent from experience in the UK that centrally-directed schemes of this type are unlikely to succeed, with the occasional exception at regional level. Also, such schemes do not easily transplant across national boundaries: a good system in London would not work in New York; a plan made for Oklahoma would not be appropriate for Saudi Arabia.

Given sufficient financial resources (which does not apply to a significant fraction of the human race) there is no reason why full radioassay services should not be available anywhere in the World. How this is achieved can be left to local decisions — to refer samples to other laboratories, or to set up a local laboratory if throughput is sufficient. In most areas simple economics and the law of supply and demand will determine the pattern. This being the case, is there any role for Government or quasi-Government involvement in the provision of assay services? Six important functions can be proposed:

(1) If no services exist, Government can provide a nucleus from which further expansion can take place (Belcher, 1978).

(2) Government can provide, or at least stimulate, screening services which are of benefit to the whole population (e.g., α-fetoprotein screening for neural tube defects).

(3) Government can provide certain basic reagents which are key to the maintenance of quality of services (distribution of standards by WHO is a good example).

(4) Government can supervise the introduction and production of 'kit' reagents, whether commercial or non-commercial (the activities of the Food and Drug Administration in the USA are a good, though not perfect, example of this).

(5) Government can and should sponsor permanent external quality control schemes (see § 11.5), with the right to advise and/or exclude laboratories which do not meet acceptable standards.

(6) Government should monitor the pricing of assay services — to avoid the situation in which an expensive research assay becomes a cheap routine test without apparent benefit to the patient.

Appendices

Appendix I

Manufacturers and suppliers of equipment

I.1. Radiation counters (automatic and/or manual sample changers)

For a classified list of commercially available well-scintillation counting systems suitable for use in radioassay see Morris and Dudley (1978).

Ames and Co.
Division of Miles Laboratories Inc.
1127 Myrtle Street, Elkhart
IN 46514, USA

Beckman Instruments Inc.
2500 Harbor, Fullerton
CA 92634, USA

ICN Pharmaceutical NV
277 Antwerpsesteenweg
B-2800 Mechelen, Belgium

Innotron Ltd.
2 Avenue Lane, Cowley Road
Oxford, OX4 1EY, U.K.

Intertechnique
Western House, 4a Hercies Road
Uxbridge, UB10 9NA, U.K.

Kontron Technik AG
Bernerstrasse 169
CH-8048 Zurich, Switzerland

Berthold Instruments
Calmbacher Strasse 22
D-7547 Wildbad 1, FRG

LKB Produkter AB
P.O. Box 76
S-16125 Stockholm 1, Sweden

Nuclear Enterprises Ltd.
Sighthill
Edinburgh, Scotland

Packard Instruments Inc.
2200 Warrenville Road
Downer's Grove
IL 60616, USA

Picker International Operations
GmbH
Seldbergstrasse 6
D-6201 Auringen, FRG

Searle Analytic Inc.
2000 Nuclear Drive, Desplaines
IL 60018, USA

Wilj Electronics Ltd.
Briscall House, Wotton Road
Ashford, Kent, U.K.

I.2. Radiation monitors

Mini-Instruments Ltd.
8 Station Industrial Estate
Burnham on Crouch, Essex, U.K.

I.3. Fluorometers

Perkin-Elmer Ltd.
Beaconsfield
Buckinghamshire, HP9 1QA, U.K.

I.4. Centrifuges

MSE Ltd.
Manor Royal
Crawley, Sussex, U.K.

Baird and Tatlock Ltd.
P.O. Box 1
Romford, Essex, U.K.

IEC
115 Fourth Ave., Boston
MA 02195, USA

Sorvall Instruments
EI Du Pont de Nemours Inc.
Instrument Products
Biomedical Division, Newton
CT 06470, USA

I.5. Pipetting apparatus (automatic/manual)

Hook and Tucker Ltd.
Vulcan Way
New Addington, U.K.

Micromedic Systems Inc.
Rohm and Haas Building
Independence Mall West
Philadelphia, PA 19105, USA

Vitatron NV
23 Spoorstraat
Dieren, The Netherlands

LKB Produkter AB
P.O. Box 76
S-161 25 Stockholm, Sweden

Eppendorf Geratebau
Postfach 324
D-2000 Hamburg 63, FRG

Oxford Laboratories
Foster City
CA 94404, USA

Labsystems Oy
Pulttitie 9
SF-00810 Helsinki 81, Finland

Scientific Manufacturing Industries
1399 64th Street, Emeryville
CA 94608, USA

Hamilton Company
P.O. Box 10030, Reno
NV 89510, USA

Centaur Sciences Inc.
Stamford
CT 06902, USA

I.6. Electrophoresis equipment

Shandon Southern Ltd.
Frimley Road
Camberley, Surrey, U.K.

Buchler Instruments Inc.
1327 16th Street, Fort Lee
NJ 07024, USA

Canal Industrial Corp.
5635 Fisher Lane, Rockville
MD 20852, USA

I.7. Automated and semi-automated systems [see review Ingrand (1978)]

Micromedic Systems Inc.
Rohm and Haas Building
Independence Mall West
Philadelphia, PA 19105, USA

LKB-Produkter, AB
P.O. Box 76
S-161 25 Stockholm 1, Sweden

Baird and Tatlock Ltd.
Chadwell Heath
Essex, U.K.

CEA
13040 Saluggia
Vercelli, Italy

Packard Instruments Inc.
2200 Warrenville Road
Downer's Grove
IL 60616, USA

Picker International Operations GmbH
Wiesbaden, Seldbergstrasse 6
D-6201 Auringen, FRG

Technicon Instruments Corp.
Tarrytown
NY 10591, USA

Union Carbide Inc.
Clinical Diagnostics
491 Theodore Fremd Avenue
Rye, NY 10580, USA

E.R. Squibb and Sons Inc.
Princeton
NJ 08540, USA

Berchtold Instruments
Calmbacher Strasse 22
D-5470 Wildbad 1, FRG

Innotron Ltd.
2 Avenue Lane
Cowley Road, Oxford, U.K.

I.8. Calculators

Hewlett-Packard Inc.
Route 41, Avondale
PA 19311, USA

Tektronix Inc.
P.O. Box 500, Beaverton
OR 97005, USA

Monroe, The Calculator Co.
The American Road, Morris Plains
NJ 07950, USA

Olivetti Corp. of America
500 Park Ave., New York
NY 10022, USA

I.9. Tubes, tube racks, etc.

Luckham Ltd.
Labro Works, Victoria Gardens
Burgess Hill, Sussex, U.K.

I.10. Columns for
chromatography

Wright Scientific Ltd.
Cardigan Road
London, NW6, U.K.

Pharmacia AB
P.O. Box 604
S-751 25 Uppsala 1, Sweden

I.11. Filtration equipment

Millipore Corp.
Bedford
MA 01730, USA

Sartorius-Membranfilter GmbH
D-3400 Gottingen, FRG

I.12. Vial openers

Identa Systems
10655 NE 4th Street
Suite 400, Bellevue
WA 98400, USA

Appendix II

Suppliers of special reagents and chemicals

II.1. General

National Pituitary Agency
Suite 5037
210 West Fayette Street, Baltimore
MD 21201, USA

Medical Research Council
Division of Biological Standards
Holly Hill Laboratories
Hampstead, London, NW3, U.K.

For lists of available Biological Standards and Reference materials see J. Endocrinol. (1979) 80, 171–174. For control sera and supplies see Radioassay News (1978) 5, 43.

II.2. Isotopes and isotopically-labelled materials

Amersham International
Amersham, Bucks, U.K.

New England Nuclear
Atomlight Place, North Billerica
MA 01862, USA

CEA/IRE/SORIN
13040 Saluggia
Vercelli, Italy

Nuclear Research Center-Negev
P.O. Box 9001
Beer-Sheva, Israel

II.3. Antisera

Antibodies Inc.
P.O. Box 442, Davis
CA 95696, USA

Calbiochem Inc.
P.O. Box 12087, San Diego
CA 92112, USA

ILS Ltd.
14–15 Newbury Street
London, EC1, U.K.

Inolex Biomedical
2600 Bond Street
Park Forest South
IL 60466, USA

Miles Laboratories
Stoke Court
Stoke Poges, Bucks, U.K.

Serono Biodata
Via Casilina 125
00176, Rome, Italy

Wellcome Reagents Ltd.
Beckenham
Kent, U.K.

II.4. Hormones

II.4.1. Human placental lactogen
ILS Ltd.
14–15 Newbury Street
London, EC1, U.K.

II.4.2. Adrenocorticotrophin ('Synacthen')
Ciba Laboratories
Horsham, Sussex, U.K.

II.4.3. Steroid hormones
Steraloids Inc.
Wilton
NH 03086, USA

II.5. Double-antibody solid phase

Organon Scientific Development Group
P.O. Box 20, Kloosterstraat 6
Oss, Holland

II.6. Glass beads

Corning Glass Works
Corning, New York, USA

II.7. Quality controls

Hyland Diagnostics
Division of Travenol Lab. Inc.
P.O. Box 2214, 3300 Hyland Ave.
Costa Mesa, CA 92626, USA

Ortho Diagnostics Inc.
Raritan
NJ 08869, USA

Dade Division
American Hospital Supply Corp.
Miami, FL 33152, USA

Appendix III

Suppliers of general reagents and materials

Armour Pharmaceutical Co. Ltd.
International Division
Hampden Park
Eastbourne, Sussex BN22 9AA, U.K.

Bayer AG
Beraus Pharma B2
Bayerwerk
D-5090 Leverkusen, FRG

Bio-rad Laboratories
32nd and Griffin Avenue
Richmond, CA 94804, USA

British Drug Houses Ltd.
Poole, Dorset, U.K.

Calbiochem Inc.
P.O. Box 12087, San Diego
CA 92112, USA

Difco Laboratories
Detroit
MI 48232, USA

Eli Lilly International
P.O. Box 32, Indianapolis
IN 4206, USA

Hopkin and Williams Ltd.
P.O. Box 1
Romford, Essex, U.K.

Jencons Ltd.
Mark Road, Hemel Hempstead
Herts, U.K.

Koch-Light Laboratories Ltd.
Colnbrook, Bucks, U.K.

Merck, E.
D-6100 Darmstadt FRG

Oxoid Ltd.
Southwark Bridge Road
London, SE1 U.K.

Pharmacia AB
P.O. Box 604
S-751 25 Uppsala 1
Sweden

Sigma Chemical Co.
P.O. Box 14508, St Louis
MO 63178, USA

Whatman Labsales Ltd.
Springfield Mill
Maidstone, Kent, U.K.

Appendix IV

Manufacturers of reagent kits for radioimmunoassay and related techniques

Note: Commercial manufacture of RIA kits is a fast moving subject, with numerous takeovers, name changes, and product line changes. Detailed information is likely to be out of date before it is printed, but a detailed list of kits and manufacturers appeared in Clinical Chemistry (1978) 24, 1223.

Abbott Laboratories
Abbott Park, North Chicago
IL 60064, USA

Ames Company
Division of Miles Laboratories, Inc.
1127 Myrtle Street, Elkhard
IN 46514, USA

Beckman Instruments Inc.
Campus Drive at Jamboree Blvd.
Irvine, CA 92664, USA

Becton Dickinson Immunodiagnostics
Mountain View Ave., Orangeburg
NY 10962, USA

Biolab
Avenue de Tervuren 142
1040 Bruxelles, Belgium

BIO-RIA, Bio-Endocrinology Inc.
10850 Hamon Street, Montreal
Quebec, Canada

Calbiochem
10933 N. Torrey Pines Road
San Diego, CA 92037, USA

Cambridge Nuclear Radio-pharma-
ceutical Corp.
575 Middlesex Turnpike, Billerica
MA 08165, USA

CEA/IRE/SORIN
13040 Saluggia
Vercelli, Italy

Clinical Assays Inc.
237 Binney Street, Cambridge
MA 02142, USA

Corning Diagnostics
Medfield
MA 02052, USA

Curtis Laboratories Inc.
1948 East 46th Street, Los Angeles
CA 90058, USA

Data Diagnostics Corp.
3401 Main Street, Houston
TX 77002, USA

Diagnostic Product Corp.
12306 Exposition Blvd., Los Angeles
CA 90064, USA

Electro-Nucleonics Laboratories Inc.
4809 Auburn Ave., Bethesda
MD 20014, USA

Endocrine Sciences
18418 Oxnard Street, Tarzana
CA 91365, USA

Fisher Scientific Co.
711 Forbes Avenue, Pittsburgh.
PA 15219, USA

General Medical Systems Inc.
3814 Cavalier Street, Garland
TX 75042, USA

International Diagnostics Technology
Santa Clara
CA 95050, USA

Interscience Institute
200 Cotner Ave., Los Angeles
CA 90052, USA

Kallestad Laboratories Inc.
100 Lake Hazeltine Drive Chaska
MN 55318, USA

Life Systems Inc.
505 Northern Blvd. Great Neck
NY 11021, USA

Mallinckrodt Inc.
75 Brown Road, Hazlewood
MO 63042, USA

Meloy Laboratories Inc.
6715 Electronic Drive, Springfield
VA 22151, USA

New England Nuclear
549 Albany Street, Boston
MA 02118, USA

Nichols Institute
1300 Beacon Street, San Pedro
CA 90731, USA

Nuclear Diagnostics Inc.
575 Robbins Drive, Troy
MI 48084, USA

Nuclear International Inc.
215 Middlesex Turnpike, Burlington
MA 01803, USA

Nuclear Medical Systems Inc.
515 Superior Avenue, Newport Beach
CA 92660, USA

Pantex
P.O. Box 966, Malibu
CA 90265, USA

Pharmacia Laboratories
P.O. Box 604
S-751 25 Uppsala 1, Sweden

Quantimetrix
P.O. Box 1693, Beverley Hills
CA 90213, USA

Radioassay Systems Laboratories Inc.
1511 E. Del Amo Blvd., Carson
CA 90746, USA

Amersham International
Amersham, Bucks, U.K.

RIA Diagnostics
8226 Allport Avenue
Santa Fe Springs
CA 90670, USA

RIA Products Inc.
P.O. Box 914
97 Beaver Street, Waltham
MA 02154, USA

Roche Diagnostics
Kingsland Street, Nutley
NJ 07011, USA

Schwartz-Mann
Mountain View Ave., Orangeburg
NY 10962, USA

Seward Laboratory
UAC House, Blackfriars Road
London SE1 9UG, U.K.

Smith Kline Instruments Inc.
880 W. Maude Ave., Sunnyville
CA 94086, USA

E.R. Squibb and Sons Inc.
P.O. Box 4000, Princeton
NJ 08540, USA

Syva Corp.
3181 Porter Drive, Palo Alto
CA 94304, USA

Union Carbide Clinical Diagnostics
401 Theodore Fremd Avenue, Rye
NY 10580, USA

Wellcome Research Laboratories
Beckenham, Kent, U.K.

Wien Laboratories Inc.
P.O. Box 27, Succasunna
NJ 07876, USA

Appendix V

Safety precautions in the handling of radioactive isotopes

Contamination of personnel with radioactive isotopes is regarded as one of the greatest hazards of work in a biomedical laboratory. As a result there are stringent regulations and requirements for precautions in the handling of these materials. Although the amounts of radioactivity involved in radioimmunoassay are relatively small such precautions must be strictly observed. A set of general rules for this type of work is presented here, which can perhaps be summarised as commonsense, care and the realisation that any errors are easily detected. A more formal account may be found in the 'Code of Practice for the Protection of Persons against Ionizing Radiations arising from Medical and Dental Use' (1972, London, Her Majesty's Stationery Office) and in 'Rules and Regulations', Title 10 —Chapter 1, Code of Federal Regulations (codified and reissued 1975, US Nuclear Regulatory Commission, Washington DC).

V.1. Radiation hazards in the RIA laboratory

There are 3 main hazards in the handling of unsealed sources of radioactivity:

(1) *External β- and γ-irradiation*:   These are of little importance in the RIA laboratory because the total amounts of radioactivity are relatively small and the γ-radiation of the principle isotope used (^{125} I) is of low energy (0.027 MeV) and has little penetration.

(2) *Skin contamination*:   This is very common and at high levels might lead to skin necrosis. More important, unrecognised contamination of the hands is likely to lead to ingestion of isotope and deposition in the body (see (3) below).

(3) *Ingestion and deposition of isotopes in the body*:   This is the major hazard, and usually arises as the result of preparation and consumption of food and beverages by personnel with unrecognised contamination of skin or clothing. ^{125} I localises in the thyroid gland in which it may, at high levels, cause acute necrosis. In the long-term, there is also a potential carcinogenic hazard.

V.2. General administration

Laboratory areas used for the handling of radioisotopes should be designated as such, and the use and storage of isotopes strictly confined to these areas. The areas should be clearly identified by the display of internationally accepted warning signs (available in the U.K. from Jencons Ltd.) In larger laboratories, further areas should be designated for the handling of bulk quantities of radioisotopes (> 1 mCi) and subjected to particularly rigorous inspection. These areas should be provided with fume cupboards for all high activity work, should be well-ventilated, and should have a shower facility against the possibility of severe skin contamination. No personnel should be permitted to work in any of these areas unless they have received instruction in the safe handling of isotopes.

Every laboratory, however small, should appoint one member of the staff as the Radiation Safety Officer (RSO) who will be responsible for instructing and advising the staff in relation to radiation protection, for periodic monitoring of both staff and equipment for contamination, and for assisting in the event of an accidental spill. The RSO is also responsible for maintaining a log of all radioactivity entering the laboratory, and for its eventual route of disposal. In most Western countries such records are a statutory requirement.

V.3. Rules for handling radioactive preparations

The following rules apply to all levels of radioactivity. High levels of activity ($>$ 1 mCi ^{125}I) should always be handled in a Class 3 laboratory (see below) with particularly stringent precautions:

(1) Laboratory coats must always be worn in the laboratories.
(2) No eating, drinking or smoking should be permitted in the active laboratories.
(3) Disposable gloves must be worn for all procedures involving solutions with radioactive concentrations $>$ 0.1 μCi/ml and large volumes of lower concentration but total activity $>$ 10 μCi.
(4) Hands must be monitored with a simple end-window radiation monitor (Mini-Instruments Ltd.) immediately after handling any activity $>$ 1 mCi, both before and after removal of gloves.
(5) All radioactive sources of concentration $>$ 0.01 μCi/ml or total content $>$ 1 μCi must be clearly labelled stating the isotope, activity, date and volume.
(6) Pipetting must *never* be performed by mouth.
(7) Disposable containers and pipetting devices with dispensible tips should be used whenever possible.
(8) All bench top areas should have disposable coverings (e.g., 'Benchkote', Whatman Labsales) which are regularly monitored and replaced as necessary.
(9) Procedures involving high levels of activity ($>$ 0.1 mCi) should be carried out in a tray which is monitored immediately after use. Where possible all glassware should be disposable. Handling of vials containing high activity should be kept as brief as possible, and lead shielding should be used where available.
(10) All non-disposable equipment (columns, syringes, pipettes) used for high levels of activity should be thoroughly rinsed in running water after use and then allowed to soak in a detergent solution

until required again. Such equipment should always be stored in the 'hot' laboratory and not taken for use outside.

(11) All tools (bottle openers, forceps etc.) should be checked for contamination before being put away.

(12) All sources of activity > 0.1 mCi should be stored in a separate and designated area, preferably with lead shielding.

V.4. Monitoring of the laboratory

All benches and equipment in low-activity laboratories should be monitored once a week, and in high activity laboratories after completion of every procedure. The permissible level of contamination is 10^{-3} μCi/cm^2 averaged over an area not greater than 300 cm^2.

V.5. Monitoring of personnel

All personnel should have a general medical examination and a full blood examination at the time of first employment. The blood examination should be repeated at yearly intervals. All working staff should be provided with a film badge which is examined and changed at monthly intervals. The maximum permissible dose level is equivalent to 5 rem*/annum to critical organs such as the gonads, bone marrow and eye, or 3 rem in any one quarter. In practice, such doses are very rare even in the busiest radioassay laboratory. Personnel working with iodine isotopes should have a thyroid count performed every month. The maximum permitted dose to this organ is 30 rem/annum, equivalent to the inhalation of 21 μCi ^{125}I. In a typical well-run laboratory exposure is only 1/1000th of this.

---

* The 'rem' is a dose equivalent derived from the absorbed dose measured in 'rad', and a quality factor and a distribution factor which depend on the type of radiation. One rad is the dose absorbed when 62.5×10^6 MeV of energy is deposited in 1 g of matter (the equivalent Systeme International Unit is the 'sievert' (Sv); 1 Sv sievert = 100 rems exactly).

V.6. Disposal of radiaoactive waste

The rules for disposal of radioactive waste vary widely both between countries and within the same country. For this reason every laboratory should consult their appropriate local authority for guidance. The amount of isotope (if any) which can be disposed of via mains drainage is determined by local regulations.

V.7. Emergency procedure for spills of radioactive materials

The RSO and Head of Department should be informed at once. No personnel should be permitted into the affected area unless wearing gloves and overshoes, both of which must be disposed of on leaving the area. Any contaminated clothing must be removed and discarded. If the spill is on the skin the area should be flushed thoroughly with tap water taking great care not to spread the contamination. Decontamination should aim at getting activity down to 10^{-4} $\mu Ci/cm^2$. Contaminated areas should be carefully mopped with disposable paper, then washed until activity is down to 10^{-4} $\mu Ci/cm^2$. If this cannot be achieved the area must be temporarily covered with polythene sheeting.

V.8. Design of radioassay laboratory

Radioassay kits, as opposed to bulk isotopes, can be handled in any general clinical laboratory (Class 3). However, their use should be confined to a specified area which is provided with appropriate warning signs and is regularly monitored for contamination. Bulk isotopes ($\geqslant 1$ mCi) should only be handled in a Class 2 radioisotope laboratory which has the following general specifications:
(1) Walls and ceilings; washable, non-porous paint.
(2) Floor: washable linoleum, rubber or vinyl; joins between floors and walls should be rounded.
(3) Sinks; connected to main drainage, stoppers and taps should be operated by foot pedal.
(4) Ventilation; air flow must be to the outside of the building or to an appropriate filter.
(5) Fume cupboards; must have an eddy-free airflow drawing at least

150 ft/min and vented to the outside of the building or to an appropriate filter. A self-contained charcoal-filter unit with 90% trapping efficiency is available from Interex Corp. (3 Strathmore Road, Natick, MA 01760, USA).

(6) Shower; a shower facility should be available immediately adjacent to the high-activity area.

Appendix VI

Commonly-used procedures for the attachment of ligands to carrier molecules or solid-phase materials

There are many situations in the development of a binding assay in which it is essential to attach one molecule to another molecule or to a solid phase. Examples include the preparation of haptens as immunogens (§ 5.2.3), the attachment of labels by indirect methods (§ 4.2), the preparation of solid phase antibodies (§ 6.3.6.2), and the preparation of solid phase antigens for use in immunometric procedures (§ 6.4). In this appendix the mechanisms of some of the commonly-used procedures are summarised; in some cases the mechanism has been simplified for the sake of clarity.

VI.1. Cyanogen bromide

Cyanogen bromide reacts with hydroxyl groups on a solid-phase polysaccharide matrix (e.g., Sepharose) to form cyclic imidocarbonates.

IMIDOCARBONATE

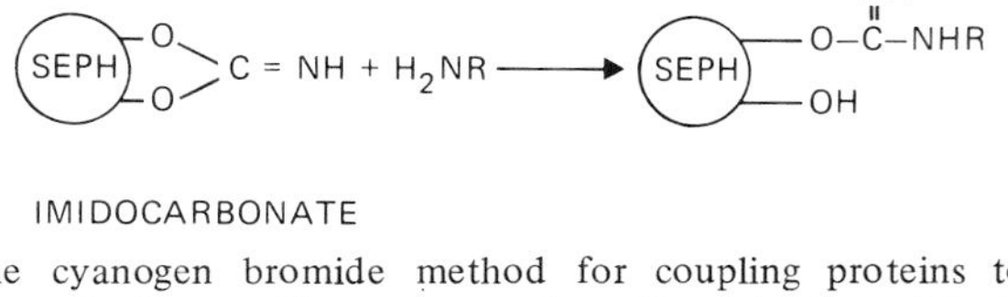

Fig. VI.1. The cyanogen bromide method for coupling proteins to insoluble matrices such as Sepharose. The cyanogen bromide activation of Sepharose leads to the formation of a cyclic imidocarbonate (shown here), which can react with amino groups on the ligand (R) to form a covalent linkage between the ligand and Sepharose.

TABLE VI.1
Preparation of a solid-phase antibody

(modified from Gardner, Bailey and Chard, 1974)

---

1. Prepare a γ-globulin fraction from the antiserum by adding 1.8 g of Na_2SO_4 (anhydrous) to 10 ml of serum, mixing for 30 min, centrifuging at 2000 x g for 10 min, washing the precipitate twice with 10 ml of 18% (w/v) Na_2SO_4, and re-dissolving in 10 ml 0.8% NaCl.
2. Swell 1 g cyanogen bromide (CNBr)-activated Sepharose 4B (Pharmacia AB) in 10 mM HCl. This should be carried out on a Buchner funnel with a grade 4 Scinta glass filter. A total of 200 ml of 10 mM HCl is added and removed in several aliquots (this removes dextran and lactose which are added to the gel to preserve activity during freeze-drying).
3. After a final wash with 0.1 M $NaHCO_3$ transfer the gel to a glass tube, add 50 ml of 0.1 M $NaHCO_3$ containing 1 ml of the γ-globulin solution from 1., and mix by vertical rotation (25 rev./min) for 24 h at room temperature.
4. Wash the resultant immunoabsorbent once with 100 ml of 1.0 M ethanolamine (pH 8.0) with continuous mixing for 2 h (this blocks any residual reactive groups on the gel). Wash with 100 ml of 0.5 M $NaHCO_3$ (pH 8.3) and then with 50 ml 0.2 M sodium acetate buffer (pH 4.0). Repeat washing sequence once more (the sharp changes in pH are the key for protein desorption). Finally wash twice with 100 ml of assay diluent shown in Table 1.2, but containing in addition 0.1% (v/v) Tween 20 (Koch-Light Laboratories Ltd.), with 30 min continuous mixing for each wash. The suspension should be stored below 8°C without freezing.

Note:

(*i*) Buffers containing amino groups (e.g., Tris) should not be used during coupling because they compete with amino groups on the ligand. For the same reason, sodium sulphate is preferred to ammonium sulphate for the initial precipitation of immunoglobulins;

(*ii*) A pH of 8–10 is chosen for coupling so that the amino groups are mainly in the unprotonated form;

(*iii*) If the net recovery of antibody activity is low this may be due to:

    (a) Loss of activity during preparation of immunoglobulins (the immunoglobulin solution should always be compared with the original antiserum);

    (b) Coupling of an excessive quantity of protein (the optimum is 5–10 mg protein/ml gel);

    (c) Multi-point attachment of the immunoglobulin to the gel (this can be reduced by pre-hydrolysis of some of the active groups, allowing the gel to stand for 4 h at pH 8.3, or incorporation of competing amino groups in the reaction mixture (e.g. Tris, ethanolamine).

These react with primary amino groups on the ligand to form a covalent bond (Fig. VI.1). Cyanogen bromide-activated Sepharose is available commercially, and a procedure for coupling it to an antibody is shown in Table VI.1.

VI.1. Carbodiimides

Carbodiimides are widely used for the formation of peptide bonds between amino and carboxyl groups on adjacent molecules (e.g., the attachment of a hapten to a protein to form an immunogen (§ 5.2.3) or the attachment of ligands to solid phase matrices (Chapman and Ratcliffe, 1982) (§ 6.4). The basic structure of a carbodiimide is:

$$RN{=}C{=}NR$$

where R is an appropriate substituent or substituents. This reacts with carboxyl groups to give:

$$\overset{\displaystyle OCOR'}{\underset{\displaystyle RNH-C{=}NR}{\mid}}$$

where R' is the structure containing the carboxyl group (e.g., the side-chains of the amino acids glutamic acid or aspartic acid). This can further react with an amino group (NH_2-R'') to give:

$$R'CONHCR'' \ + \ RHNCONHR \ \text{(urea derivative)}$$

where R'' is the structure containing the amino group. As a result R' and R'' are now linked by a peptide bond, and a urea derivative is formed. It is desirable that the carbodiimide and the urea derivative should be water-soluble, and two water-soluble carbodiimides are in common use:

1-ethyl-3-(3-dimethyl-amino-propyl) carbodiimide hydrochloride (EDC):

$$CH_3-CH_2-N{=}C{=}N-CH_2-CH_2-CH_2-N^+(CH_3)_2Cl^-$$

and

1 -cyclohexyl-3 -(2 -morpholino-ethyl) carbodiimide metho-p-toluene sulphonate (CMC).

Both EDC and CMC can be obtained through most suppliers of general biochemicals. A typical procedure for coupling a hapten to a protein carrier is shown in Table VI.2.

TABLE VI.2
Procedure for coupling a hapten to a protein using carbodiimides

The hapten can be any small molecule containing carboxyl or amino groups (e.g., a peptide or an appropriately modified steroid)

1. Dissolve 100 mg of bovine serum albumin in distilled water (see note (*i*), below).
2. Add sufficient ligand so that there are approximately 20–40 molecules of ligand to each molecule of albumin.
3. Slowly add 200 mg of the carbodiimide EDC (see p. 264) with constant mixing; check the pH continuously during the addition and add small amounts of 1 N HCl as necessary to keep the pH close to 5.5.
4. Allow the reaction to continue for 4–12 h with continuous checks on pH and adjustment to pH 5.5 if necessary.
5. Dilute the mixture with 10 ml distilled water and dialyse for 24 h at 4°C against several changes of distilled water or an appropriate buffer.
6. Store the product in aliquots at −20°C.

Note:

(*i*) The volumes used should be as small as possible given the need to introduce a stirring bar and a pH electrode;
(*ii*) The concentration of carbodiimide should be 10 to 100 times that of the coupled spacer groups;
(*iii*) The carbodiimide should be as fresh as possible;
(*iv*) All steps except for final dialysis are carried out at room temperature;
(*v*) Precipitation may occur during the reaction due to the formation of cross links between albumin molecules − this does not indicate that the reaction is unsuccessful. Precipitation may also occur during dialysis because of insolubility of the final product;
(*vi*) It is good practice to monitor the efficiency of the conjugation by incorporating a small amount of tracer ligand in the system. Alternatively, the efficiency of steroid coupling can be assessed by measuring the ultraviolet spectrum of the conjugate (Erlanger et al., 1958);
(*vii*) If the ligand is not readily soluble in water an organic solvent such as dioxane or dimethylformamide at up to 50% is used

VI.3. Diisocyanates

Diisocyanates can be used to link adjacent amino-groups. Phenylene diisothiocyanate has the structure:

$$S=C=N \overset{N=C=S}{}$$

The isothiocyanate group can react with a primary amine to form a covalent bond:

$$R-NH_2 + S=C=N-R' \rightarrow R-\underset{H}{N}-\underset{S}{\overset{\parallel}{C}}-\underset{H}{N}-R'$$

and a diisothyiocyanate can therefore serve to link amino groups on adjacent molecules.

VI.4. Aldehydes

The most familiar of these is glutaraldehyde (Avrameas, 1969):

$$(CH_3)_3 \overset{CHO}{\underset{CHO}{\diagdown}}$$

The aldehyde groups can each react with primary amines to form covalent bonds:

$$R-NH_2 + O=\overset{H}{\underset{}{C}}-R' \rightarrow R-N=\overset{H}{\underset{}{C}}-R' + H_2O$$

and thus link adjacent molecules.

VI.5. The mixed anhydride reaction

The ligand (e.g., a carboxymethyloxime derivative of a steroid) is reacted with isobutyl chloroformate in non-aqueous solvent to form a mixed anhydride (Erlanger et al., 1959):

$$R-COOH + R'COCl \longrightarrow \begin{array}{c} RCO \\ \diagdown \\ O \\ \diagup \\ R'CO \end{array} + HCl$$

where R–COOH is the steroid carboxymethyloxime, and R′COCl is isobutyl chloroformate. The mixture includes tri-n-butylamine which acts as a weak base to 'mop up' the HCl formed. The mixed anhydride can then react with primary amino groups of a protein in an alkaline aqueous solution:

$$\begin{array}{c} RCO \\ \diagdown \\ O \\ \diagup \\ R'CO \end{array} + R''NH_2 \longrightarrow RCO-HNR'' + R'COOH$$

Because the mixed anhydride is formed prior to reaction with the protein this procedure does not lead to the formation of cross-linked, insoluble protein molecules. A typical procedure is shown in Table VI.3.

VI.6. m-Maleimidobenzyl-N-hydroxysuccinimide ester (MBS)

This is the best known of the so-called 'hetero-bifunctional' reagents. The linkage proceeds by two separate reactions, thus avoiding formation of bonds between identical molecules. MBS has the structure:

TABLE VI.3
Procedure for linking a hapten to a protein by a mixed anhydride reaction
(preparation of oestriol-6-BSA)

1. Dissolve 50 mg of oestriol-6-carboxymethyloxime (Steraloids Inc.) in 10 ml dioxane.
2. Add 0.1 ml tri-n-butylamine.
3. Cool the solution to 10°C, add 0.02 ml isobutyl-chloroformate and stir for 30 min.
4. Dissolve 100 mg of crystalline grade bovine serum albumin (Sigma Chemical Co.) in 10 ml distilled water adjusted to pH 9 with 2 M NaOH.
5. Mix the two solutions and stir at 4°C for 24 h.
6. Dialyse the reaction mixture against water for 36 h.
7. Freeze-dry the solution (conjugate) remaining in the dialysis bag.

Under appropriate conditions this reacts by both acylation of amino-groups via the active *N*-hydroxyester and formation of thioether bonds by addition of a thiol to the double bond of the maleimide. MBS has been used for the conjugation of enzymes to protein hormones for enzyme immunoassay (Kitagawa and Aikawa, 1976).

References

Abraham, G.E. (1969) J. Clin. Endocrinol, Metab. *29*, 2866.

Addison, G.M. and Hales, C.N. (1971) Horm. Res. *3*, 59.

Aherne, G.W., Marks, V., Mould, G. and Stout, G. (1977) Lancet *i*, 1214.

Al-Dujaili, E.A.S., Forrest, G.C., Edwards, C.R.W. and Landon, J. (1979) Clin. Chem. *25*, 1402.

Anderson, D.C. (1970) Clin. Chim. Acta *29*, 513.

Andrieu, J., Manas, S. and Dray, F. (1975) in: Steroid Immunoassay (Cameron, E., Hillier, S. and Griffiths, K. eds) p. 189, Alpha-Omega-Alpha, Cardiff.

Apinyacharti, P. and Baxter, R.C. (1979) Clin. Chem. *25*, 161.

Arquilla, E.R. and Stavitsky, A.B. (1956) J. Clin. Invest. *35*, 458.

Atassi, M.Z. (1978) Immunochemistry *15*, 909.

Avrameas, S. (1969) Immunochemistry *6*, 43.

Axelsson, B., Eriksson, H., Borrebaeck, C., Mattiasson, B. and Sjögren, H.O. (1981) J. Immunol. Methods *41*, 351.

Bagshawe, K.D. (1975) Lab. Prac. 573.

Bangham, D.R. and Cotes, P.M. (1974) Brit. Med. Bull. *30*, 12.

Barisas, B.G., Singer, S.J. and Sturtevant, J.M. (1977) Immunochemistry *14*, 247.

Beckers, C., Cornette, C., Francois, B., Bouckaert, A. and Lechat, M. (1978) in: Radioimmunoassay and Related Procedures in Medicine 1977, vol. II, p. 341, International Atomic Energy Agency, Vienna.

Belanger, L., Sylvestre, C. and Dufour, D. (1973) Clin. Chim. Acta *48*, 15.

Belcher, E.M. (1978) Atomic Energy Rev. *16*, 485.

Belchetz, P.E. (1976) Proc. Roy. Soc. Med. *69*, 428.

Benson, R.C., Riggs, B.L., Pickard, B.M. and Arnaud, C. (1974) J. Clin. Invest. *54*, 175.

Berson, S.A. and Yalow, R.S. (1969) Science *152*, 205.

Berson, S.A., Yalow, R.S., Bauman, A., Rothschild, M.A. and Newerly, K. (1956) J. Clin. Invest. *35*, 170.

Binoux, M.A. and Odell, S.E. (1973) J. Clin. Endocr. Metab. *36*, 303.

Birnbaumer, L. and Pohl, S.L. (1973) J. Biol. Chem. *248*, 2056.

Blake, C.C.F. (1975) Nature *253*, 158.

Blanchard, G.C. and Gardner, R. (1978) Clin. Chem. *24*, 808.

Bloom, S. (1974) Brit. Med. Bull. *30*, 62.

Boitieux, J.-L., Desnet, G. and Thomas, D. (1979) Clin. Chem. *25*, 318.

Bolton, A.E. and Hunter, W.M. (1973) Biochem. J. *133*, 529.

Boyd, G.W., Landon, J. and Peart, W.S. (1967) Lancet *ii*, 1002.

Brooker, G., Terasaki, W.L. and Price, M.G. (1976) Science *194*, 270.

Broughton, A. and Strong, J.E. (1976) Clin. Chim. Acta *66*, 125.

Broughton, A., Strong, J.E., Pickering, L.K., Knight, J. and Bodey, G.P. (1978) Clin. Chem. *24*, 717.

Brown, T.R., Bagchi, N., Ho, T.T.S. and Mack, R.E. (1980) Clin. Chem. *26*, 503.

Bundesen, P.G., Drake, R.G., Kelly, K., Worsley, I.G., Friesen, H.G. and Sehon, A.H. (1980) J. Clin. Endocr. Metab. *51*, 1472.

Burd, J.F., Carrico, R.J., Fetter, M.C., Buckler, R.T., Johnson, R.D., Boguslaski, R.C. and Christner, J.E. (1977) Anal. Biochem. *77*, 56.

Butt, W.R. (1972) J. Endocrinol. *55*, 453.

Buttner, J., Borth, R., Boutwell, J.H. and Broughton, P.M.G. (1975) Clin. Chim. Acta *63*, F25.

Cais, M., Dani, S., Edden, Y., Gandolfi, O., Horn, M., Isaacs, E.E., Josephy, Y., Saar, Y., Slovin, E. and Snarsky, L. (1977) Nature 270, 534.

Cambiaso, C.L., Leek, A.E., De Steenwinkel, F., Billen, J. and Masson, P.L. (1977) J. Immunol. Methods *18*, 33.

Catt, K.J. and Tregear, C.W. (1967) Science *158*, 1570.

Catt, K.J., Dufau, M.L. and Tsuruhara, T. (1972) J. Clin. Endocr. Metab. *34*, 123.

Challand, G.S., Goldie, D.J. and Landon, J. (1974) Brit. Med. Bull. *30*, 38.

Challand, G.W., Spencer, C.A. and Ratcliffe, J.G. (1976) Ann. Clin. Biochem. *13*, 354.

Chapman, R.S. and Ratcliffe, J.G. (1982) Clin. Chim. Acta *118*, 129.

Chard, T. (1971) *in*: Radioimmunoassay Methods (Kirkham, K.E. and Hunter, W.M. eds) p. 491, Churchill Livingstone, Edinburgh, London.

Chard, T. and Sykes, A. (1979) Clin. Chem. *25*, 973.

Chard, T., Kitau, M.J. and Landon, J. (1970) J. Endocrinol. *46*, 269.

Chard, T., Martin, M.J. and Landon, J. (1971) *in*: Radioimmunoassay Methods (Kirkham, K.E. and Hunter, W.M. eds) p. 257, Churchill Livingstone, Edinburgh, London.

Chen, I.-W., Heminger, L., Maxon, H.R. and Tsay, J.Y. (1980) Clin. Chem. *124*, 1551.

Chopra, I.J. (1972) J. Clin. Endocrinol. *34*, 938.

Clapp, J.J. (1978) Radioassay News *5*, 53.

Cocola, F., Orlandi, A., Barbarulli, G., Tarli, P. and Neri, P. (1979) Anal. Biochem. *99*, 121.

Collins, W.P. and Hennan, J.F. (1976) Mol. Asp. Med. *1*, 1.

Cornish-Bowden, A. and Koshland, D.E. (1975) J. Mol. Biol. *95*, 201.

Creese, I. and Snyder, S.M. (1977) Nature *270*, 180.

Curry, R.E., Heitzman, H., Riege, D.H., Sweet, R.V. and Simonsen, M.G. (1979) Clin. Chem. *25*, 1591.

Dandliker, W.B., Hicks, A.N., Levison, S.A. and Brawn, R.J. (1977) Biochem. Biophys. Res. Commun. *74*, 538.

Dandliker, W.B., Kelly, R.G., Dandliker, J., Farquhar, J. and Levin, J. (1973) Immunochemistry *10*, 219.

Das, R.E.G. (1980) Clin. Chem. *26*, 1726.

Dawes, C.C. and Gardner, J. (1978) Clin. Chim. Acta *86*, 353.

Dean, P.D.G., Exley, D. and Johnson, M.W. (1971) Steroids *18*, 543.

Deelder, A.M. and Ploem, J.S. (1974) J. Immunol. Methods *4*, 239.

Den Hollander, F.C. and Schuurs, A.H.W.M. (1971) *in*: Radioimmunoassay Methods (Kirkham, K.E. and Hunter, W.M. eds) p. 419, Churchill Livingstone, Edinburgh, London.

Dermody, W.C., Levy, A.G., Davis, P.E. and Plowman, J.K. (1979) Clin. Chem. *25*, 989.

Desbuquois, B. and Aurbach, G.D. (1971) J. Clin. Endocr. Metab. *33*, 732.

Di Bella, F.P., Kehrwald, J.M., Laskso, K. and Zitsner, L. (1978) Clin. Chem. *24*, 451.

Donini, S. and Donini, P. (1969) Acta Endocrinol. København) Suppl. *142*, 257.

Dotti, C., Becchi, A., Castagnetti, C., Colla, B. and Fillipi, G. (1979) Steroids *33*, 527.

Dyas, J., Turkes, A., Read, G.F. and Riad-Famay, D. (1981) Ann. Clin. Biochem. *18*, 37.

Eisenthal, R. and Cornish-Bowden, A. (1974) Biochem. J. *139*, 715.

Ekeke, G.I., Exley, D. and Abuknesha, R. (1979) J. Steroid Biochem. *11*, 1597.

Ekins, R.P. (1960) Clin. Chim. Acta *5*, 453.

Ekins, R.P. (1969) *in*: Protein and Polypeptide Hormones (Margoulies, M. ed.) p. 633, Excerpta Medica/Elsevier, Amsterdam, New York.

Ekins, R.P. (1974) Brit. Med. Bull. *30*, 3.

Ekins, R.P. (1978) *in*: Radioimmunoassay and Related Procedures in Medicine, 1977, vol. II, p. 39, International Atomic Energy Agency, Vienna.

Ekins, R.P., Sufi, S. and Malan, P.G. (1978) *in*: Radioimmunoassay and Related Procedures in Medicine 1977, Vol. I, p. 437, International Atomic Energy Agency, Vienna.

Ekins, R.P. (1980) Nature *284*, 14.

Endres, D.B., Painter, J. and Niswender, G.D. (1978) Clin. Chem. *24*, 460.

England, B.G., Niswender, G.D. and Midgley, A.R. (1974) J. Clin. Endocr. Metab. *38*, 42.

Engvall, E. and Perlmann, P. (1971) Immunochemistry *8*, 871.

Eriksson, H., Mattiasson, B. and Thorell, J.I. (1981) J. Immunol. Methods *42*, 105.

Erlanger, B.F., Borek, G., Beiser, S.M. and Lieberman, S. (1958) J. Biol. Chem. *228*, 713.

Erlanger, B.F., Borek, G., Beiser, S.M. and Lieberman, S. (1959) J. Biol. Chem. *234*, 1090.

Eshhar, Z., Kim, J.B., Barnard, G., Collins, W.P., Gilad, S., Lindner, H.R. and Kohen, F. (1981) Steroids *38*, 89.

Feldman, H., Rodbard, D. and Levine, D. (1972) Anal. Biochem. *45*, 530.

Fischer, L. (1971) An Introduction to Gel Chromatography (Work, T.W. and Work, E. eds) Lab. Tech. Biochem. Mol. Biol. vol. 1, pt II, Elsevier Biomedical, Amsterdam, New York.

Flatt, P.R. (1980) Med. Lab. Sci. *37*, 175.

Forrest, G.C. (1977) Ann. Clin. Biochem. *14*, 1.

Fraker, F.J. and Speck, J.C. (1978) Biochem. Biophys. Res. Commun *80*, 849.

Franchimont, P. (1971) *in*: Radioimmunoassay Methods (Kirkham, K.E. and Hunter, W.M. eds) p. 535, Churchill Livingstone, Edinburgh, London.

Freedlender, A. and Cathou, R.E. (1971) *in:* Radioimmunoassay Methods (Kirkham, K. and Hunter, W.M. eds) p. 94, Churchill Livingstone, Edinburgh, London.

Frenkel, E.P., Keller, S. and McCall, M.S. (1966) J. Lab. Clin. Med. *68*, 510.

Frohman, M.A., Frohman, L.A., Goldman, M.B. and Goldman, J.N. (1979) J. Lab. Clin. Med. *93*, 614.

Fruchart, D.B., Desrumeaux, C., Denailly, P., Sezille, G., Jaillard, J., Carlier, Y., Bout, D. and Capron, A. (1978) Clin. Chem. *24*, 455.

Gable, C.A. and Shapiro, B.M. (1978) Anal. Biochem. *86*, 396.

Galen, R.S. and Forman, D. (1977) Clin. Chem. *23*, 119.

Gardner, J., Bailey, G. and Chard, T. (1974) Biochem. J. *137*, 469.

Gartner, R., Kewenig, M., Horn, K. and Scriba, P.C. (1980) J. Clin. Chem. Clin. Biochem. *18*, 571.

Gianturco, S.H., Hong, K.-Y., Steiner, M.R., Taunton, O.D., Jackson, R.L., Gotto, A.M. and Smith, L.C. (1979) Anal. Biochem. *92*, 74.

Gibbens, I., Hanlon, T.M., Skold, C.N., Russell, M.E. and Ullman, E.F. (1981) Clin. Chem. *27*, 1602.

Gibson, R.G., Hirschowitz, B.I. and Mihas, A.A. (1977) Clin. Chem. *23*, 1046.

Giese, J. and Neilsen, M.D. (1971) *in*: Radioimmunoassay Methods (Kirkham, K.E. and Hunter, W.M. eds) p. 341, Churchill Livingstone, Edinburgh, London.

Gilman, A.G. (1970) Proc. Natl. Acad. Sci. USA *67*, 305.

Givas, J.K. and Gutcho, S. (1975) Clin. Chem. *21*, 427.

Goodman, J.W. (1975) *in*: The Antigens (Sela, M. ed.) p. 127, Academic Press, New York.

Gordon, Y.B., Martin, M.J., McNeile, A.T. and Chard, T. (1973) Lancet *ii*, 1168.

Grant, D.B. (1968) Acta Endocrinol. (København) *59*, 139.

Greaves, R.I.N. (1968) Cryobiology *5*, 76.

Green, I., Paul, W.E. and Benacerraf, B. (1969) Proc. Natl. Acad. Sci. USA *64*, 1095.

Greenwood, F.C., Hunter W.M. and Glover, J.S. (1963) Biochem. J. *89*, 114.

Grenier, J., Strauss, N. and Scholler, R. (1978) *in*: Radioimmunoassay and Related Procedures in Medicine 1977, vol. I, p. 91, International Atomic Energy Agency, Vienna.

Grodsky, G.M. and Forsham, P.H. (1960) J. Clin. Invest. *39*, 1070.

Haber, E., Page, L.B. and Richards, F.F. (1965) Anal. Biochem. *12*, 163.

Haimovich, J. and Sela, M. (1966) J. Immunol. *97*, 338.

Hales, C.N. and Randle, P.J. (1963) Biochem. J. *88*, 137.

273

Hales, C.N., Beck, P., Evans, M.J. and Woodhead, J.S. (1975) *in*: Radioimmunoassay in Clinical Biochemistry (Pasternak, C.A. ed) p. 283, London, Heyden.

Halpern, E.P. and Bordens, R.W. (1979) Clin. Chem. *25*, 860.

Hammond, G.L., Ruokonen, A., Konturi, M., Koskela, E. and Vihko, R. (1977) J. Clin. Endocrin. Metab. *45*, 16.

Harris, C.C., Holken, R.H., Kookan, H. and Hsu, I.C. (1979) Proc. Natl. Acad. Sci. USA *76*, 5336.

Harrison, L.C., Flier, J., Itin, A., Kahn, C.R. and Roth, J. (1979) Science *203*, 544.

Hasler, M.J., Painter, K. and Niswender, G.D. (1975) Clin. Chem. *22*, 1850.

Hatch, K.F., Coles, E., Busey, H. and Goldman, S.C. (1976) Clin. Chem. *22*, 1383.

Healy, M.J.R. (1972) Biochem. J. *130*, 207.

Healy, M.J.R. (1979) Clin. Chem. *25*, 675.

Heber, D., Odell, W.D., Schedewie, H. and Wolfsen, A.R. (1978) Clin. Chem. *24*, 796.

Heding, L.G. (1966) *in*: Labelled Proteins in Tracer Studies (Donato, L., Milhaud, G. and Sirchis, J. eds) p. 345, European Atomic Energy Commission , Brussels.

Herbert, V., Lau, K.S., Gottlieb, C.W. and Bleicher, S.J. (1965) J. Clin. Endocr. Metab. *25*, 1375.

Hercules, D.M. and Sheehan, T.L. (1978) Anal. Chem. *50*, 22.

Hersh, L.S., Vann, W.P. and Wilhelm, S.A. (1979) Anal. Biochem. *93*, 267.

Hertl, W. and Odstrchel, G. (1978) Molec. Immunol. *16*, 173.

Hesch, R.D., Gatz, J., McIntosh, C.H.S., Jansyn, J. and Herrmann, R. (1976) Clin. Chim. Acta *70*, 33.

Hunter, W.M. (1971) *in*: Radioimmunoassay Methods (Kirkham, K.E. and Hunter, W.M. eds) p. 3, Churchill Livingstone, Edinburgh, London.

Hunter, W.M. (1978) *in*: Tumour Markers: Determination and Clinical Role (Griffiths, K., Neville, A.M. and Pierrepoint, C.G. eds) pp. 240–246, Alpha-Omega-Alpha, Cardiff.

Hunter, W.M. and Bennie, J.G. (1979) J. Endocrinol. *80*, 59.

Hunter, W.M. and Greenwood, F.C. (1964) Biochem. J. *91*, 43.

Hunter, W.M. and McKenzie, I. (1978) J. Endocrinol. *79*, 49P.

Hunter, W.M. and Budd, P.S. (1980) Lancet *ii*, 136.

Hunter, W.M. and Budd, P.S. (1981) J. Immunol. Methods *45*, 255.

Hurn, B.A. and Landon, J. (1971) *in*: Radioimmunoassay Methods (Kirkham, K.E. and Hunter, W.M. eds) p. 121, Churchill Livingstone, Edinburgh, London.

Hurwitz, E., Dietrich, F.M. and Sela, M. (1970) Eur. J. Biochem. *17*, 273.

Hwang, P., Guyda, H. and Friesen, H. (1971) Proc. Natl. Acad. Sci. USA *68*, 1902.

Ichihara, K., Yamamoto, T., Azukisawa, M. and Miyna, K. (1979) Clin. Chim. Acta *98*, 87.

Ingrand, J. (1978) Radioimmunoassay and Related Procedures in Medicine 1977, p. 185, International Atomic Energy Authority, Vienna.

Irvine, C.H.G. (1974) J. Clin. Endocr. Metab. *38*, 655.

Ismail, A.A.A., West, P.M. and Goldie, D.J. (1978) Clin. Chem. *24*, 571.

Ithakissios, D.S., Kubiatowicz, D.O. and Wicks, J.H. (1980) Clin. Chem. *26*, 323.

Jacoby, B. and Bagshawe, K.D. (1972) Cancer Res. *32*, 2413.

James, M.A.R., Chard, T. and Forsling, M.L. (1971) *in*: Radioimmunoassay Methods (Kirkham, K.E. and Hunter, W.M. eds) p. 545, Churchill Livingstone, Edinburgh, London.

Jeffcoate, S.L. (1978) *in*: Radioimmunoassay and Related Procedures in Medicine 1977, vol. II, p. 213, International Atomic Energy Agency, Vienna.

Jeffcoate, S.L. (1970) J. Steroid Biochem. *11*, 1051.

Jeffcoate, S.L. and Das, R.E.G. (1977) Ann. Clin. Biochem. *14*, 258.

Johannson, E.D.B. (1969) Acta Endocrinol. (København) *61*, 607.

Johnson, E.G., Stoneycypher, T.E. and Sturgis, B.E. (1976) Clin. Chem. *22*, 1164.

Jolley, M.E., Stroupe, S.D. and Wang, C.J. (1981) Clin. Chem. *27*, 1190.

Jonsson, S. (1978) *in*: Radioimmunoassay and Related Procedures in Medicine 1977, vol. I, p. 161, International Atomic Energy Agency, Vienna.

Jonsson, S. and Kronvall, G. (1972) Scand. J. Immunol. *1*, 414.

Joshi, U., Raghavan, V., Zemse, G., Sheth, A., Borkar, P.S. and Ramachandran, S. (1978) *in*: Enzyme Labelled Immunoassay of Hormones and Drugs (Pal, S.B. ed) p. 233, Walter de Gruyter, Berlin.

Joyce, B.C., Read, G.F. and Riad-Rahmy, D. (1978) *in*: Radioimmunoassay and Related Procedures in Medicine 1977, vol. I, p. 289, International Atomic Energy Agency, Vienna.

Jurjens, H., Pratt, J.J. and Woldring, M.G. (1975) J. Clin. Endocrinol. Metab. *40*, 19.

Kagen, L., Scheidt, S. and Roberts, L. (1975) Amer. J. Med. *58*, 177.

Kameda, N., Harte, R.A. and Deindoerfer, F.H. (1976) Clin. Chem. *22*, 1200.

Kamel, R.S., Landon, J. and Smith, D.S. (1979) Clin. Chem. *25*, 1997.

Kamel, R.S., McGregor, A.R., Landon, J. and Smith, D.S. (1979) Clin. Chim. Acta *89*, 93.

Karonen, S.-L., Morsky, P., Siren, M. and Seuderling, U. (1975) Anal. Biochem. *67*, 1.

Kato, N., Naruse, H., Irie, M. and Tsuji, A. (1979) Anal. Biochem. *96*, 419.

Keane, P.M., Walker, W.H.C., Gauldie, J. and Abraham, G.E. (1976) Clin. Chem. *22*, 70.

Kitagawa, T. and Aikawa, T. (1976) J. Biochem. *79*, 233.

Kobayashi, Y., Amitani, K., Watanabe, F. and Miyai, K. (1979) Clin. Chim. Acta *92*, 241.

Kohen, F., Hollander, Z. and Boguslaski, R.C. (1979) J. Steroid Biochem. *11*, 161.

Kohler, G. and Milstein, C. (1976) Eur. J. Immunol. *6*, 511.

Kolhouse, J.F., Kondo, H., Allen, N.C., Podell, E. and Allen, R.H. (1978) New Engl. J. Med. *299*, 785.

Korenman, S.G. (1968) J. Clin. Endocr. Metab. *28*, 127.

Krohn, K.A., Knight, L.C., Harwig, J.F. and Welch, M.J. (1977) Biochim. Biophys. Acta *490*, 497.

Kruse, V. (1979) Scand. J. Clin. Lab. Invest. *39*, 533.

Kubasik, N.P. and Sine, H.E. (1978) Clin. Chem. *24*, 137.

Kubiatowicz, D.O., Ithakissios, D.S. and Windorski, D.C. (1977) Clin. Chem. 23, 1077.

Kuss, E., Dirr, W., Goebel, R., Gloning, K., Hötzinger, H., Link, M. and Thoma, H. (1978) in: Radioimmunoassay and Related Procedures in Medicine 1977, vol. I, p. 69, International Atomic Energy Agency, Vienna.

Lader, S.R. (1978) in: Radioimmunoassay and Related Procedures in Medicine 1977, vol. I, p. 177, International Atomic Energy Agency, Vienna.

Landesman, R. and Saxena, B. (1976) Fertil. Steril. 27, 357.

Landon, J., Carney, J. and Langley, D. (1977) Ann. Clin. Biochem. 14, 90.

Langone, J.J. (1978) J. Immunol. Methods 24, 269.

Larsen, P.R. and Broskin, K. (1975) Pediatr. Res. 9, 604.

Lauzon, S. de, Cittanova, N., Desfosses, B. and Jayle, M.F. (1967) Steroids 22, 747.

Le Bouvier, G. (1972) in: Hepatitis and Blood Transfusions (Vyas, G.N., Perkins, H.A. and Schmid, R. eds) p. 97, Grune and Stratton, New York.

Lee, C.K., Killian, C.S., Murphy, G.P. and Chu, T.M. (1980) Clin. Chim. Acta 101, 209.

Lefkowitz, R.J., Roth, J. and Pastan, J. (1970) Science 170, 622.

Leonard, J.P. and Beckers, C. (1975) J. Nucl. Med. Biol. 2, 89.

Leute, R., Ullman, E.F. and Goldstein, A. (1972) J. Amer. Med. Assoc. 221, 1231.

Leuvering, J.H.W., Thal, P.J.H.M., Van der Waart, M. and Schuurs, A.H.W.M. (1980) J. Immunoassay 1, 77.

Levine, L. and Gutierrez-Cernosek, R.M. (1972) Prostaglandins 2, 281.

Levy, R.P., Marshall, J.S. and Velayo, N.L. (1971) J. Clin. Endocr. Metab. 32, 372.

Lidofsky, S.D., Imasaka, T. and Zare, R.N. (1979) Anal. Chem. 51, 1602.

Llewellyn, D.E.H., Hillier, S.G. and Read, G.F. (1977) Steroids 29, 417.

Logue, F.C., McElwee, G., Beastall, G.H. and Ratcliffe, J.G. (1978) Ann. Clin. Biochem. 15, 123.

Lynn, M. (1975) in: Enzymology (Weetall, H.H. ed) vol. 1, p. 1, Marcel Dekker, New York.

Maciejko, J.J. and Mao, S.J.T. (1982) Clin. Chem. 28, 199.

Maguire, K.P., Burrows, G.D., Norman, T.R. and Scoggins, B.A. (1978) Clin. Chem. 24, 549.

Maiolini, R., Ferrua, B. and Masseyeff, F. (1975) J. Immunol. Methods 6, 355.

Maiolini, R. and Masseyeff, F. (1975) J. Immunol. Methods 8, 223.

Malan, P.G., Cox, M.G., Long, E.M.R. and Ekins, R.P. (1978) Ann. Clin. Biochem. 15, 132.

Marana, R., Suginami, H., Robertson, D.M. and Diczfalusy, E. (1979) Acta Endocrinol. (København) 92, 585.

Marchalonis, J.J. (1969) Biochem. J. 113, 299.

Marschner, I., Erhardt, F. and Scriba, P.C. (1973) in: Radioimmunoassay and Related Procedures in Medicine, p. 111, International Atomic Energy Agency, Vienna.

Marschner, I., Erhardt, F., Henner, J. and Scriba, P.C. (1975) Z. Klin. Chem. Klin. Biochem. 13, 481.

Martin, M.J. and Landon, J. (1975) *in*: Radioimmunoassay in Clinical Biochemistry (Pasternak, C.A. ed) p. 269, Heyden, London.

Massaglia, A., Rolleri, E., Barbieri, U. and Rosa, U. (1974) J. Clin. Endocr. Metab. *38*, 820.

Mattiasson, B. (1980) J. Immunol. Methods *35*, 137.

Mattiasson, B., Svensson, K., Borrebaeck, C., Jonsson, S. and Kronvall, G. (1978) Clin. Chem. *24*, 1770.

McFarlane, A.S. (1958) Nature *182*, 53.

McGuire, W.L. (1973) J. Clin. Invest. *52*, 73.

Medhi, S.Q. (1975) *in*: Radioimmunoassay in Clinical Biochemistry (Pasternak, C.A. ed) p. 213, Heyden, London.

Meinert, C.N. and McHugh, R.B. (1968) Math. Biosci. *2*, 319.

Meriadec, B., Jolu, J.-P. and Henry, R. (1979) Clin. Chem. *25*, 1596.

Miles, L.E.M. and Hales, C.N. (1968) Nature *219*, 186.

Milstein, C. and Kohler, G. (1977) *in*: Antibodies in Human Diagnosis and Therapy (Haber, E. and Krause, R.M. eds) p. 271, Raven Press, New York.

Mitchell, M.L. and Byron, J. (1967) Diabetes *16*, 656.

Mitchell, M.L., Harden, A.B. and O'Rourke, M.E. (1960) J. Clin. Endocr. Metab. *20*, 1474.

Miyachi, Y., Vaitukaitis, J.L., Nieschlag, E. and Lipsett, M.B. (1972) J. Clin. Endocr. Metab. *34*, 23.

Miyai, K., Ishibashi, K. and Kumahara, Y. (1976) Clin. Chim. Acta *67*, 263.

Morgan, C.R. and Lazarow, W.A. (1963) Diabetes *12*, 115.

Morgan, C.R., Sorenson, R.L. and Lazarow, A. (1964) Diabetes *13*, 1 and 579.

Morris, A.C. and Dudley, R.A. (1978) *in*: Radioimmunoassay and Related Procedures in Medicine (1977) vol. I, p. 457, International Atomic Energy Agency, Vienna.

Morris, D.L., Ellis, P.B., Carrico, R.J., Yeager, F.M., Schroeder, H.R., Albarella, J.P., Boguslaski, R.C., Hornby, W.E. and Rawson, D. (1981) Anal. Chem. *53*, 658.

Morton, J.J. and Riegger, A.J.G. (1978) J. Endocrinol. *77*, 277.

Murphy, B.E.P. (1965) J. Lab. Clin. Med. *66*, 161.

Murphy, B.E.P. (1971) Nature *232*, 21.

Murphy, B.E.P., Engelberg, W. and Pattee, C.J. (1963) J. Clin. Endocr. Metab. *23*, 293.

Nargessi, R.D., Landon, J., Pourfarzaneh, M. and Smith, D.S. (1978) Clin. Chim. Acta *89*, 455.

Nargessi, R.D., Landon, J. and Smith, D.S. (1979) J. Immunol. Methods *26*, 307.

Nargessi, R.D., Ackland, J., Hassam, M., Forrest, G.C., Smith, D.S. and Landon, J. (1980) Clin. Them. *26*, 1701.

Neurath, A.R. and Strick, N. (1979) Mol. Immunol. *16*, 625.

Nielsen, S.T., Barrett, P.Q., Neumann, M.W. and Neumann, W.F. (1979) Anal. Biochem. *92*, 67.

Nieschlag, E. (1975) Immunization with Hormones in Reproduction Research, Elsevier Biomedical, Amsterdam, New York.

Nishi, S. and Hirai, H. (1975) Protides Biol. Fluids. Proc. Collq. *23*, 303.

Nisula, B.C., Ayala, A.R., Stolk, M.D., Talidouras, G.S. and Stolk, J.M. (1978) *in*: Radioimmunoassay and Related Procedures in Medicine 1977, vol. I, p. 133, International Atomic Energy Agency, Vienna.

Niswender, G.D. (1980) Ligand Rev. *2*, 70.

Nordblom, G.D., Webb, R., Counsell, R.E. and England, B.C. (1981) Steroids *38*, 161.

Nye, L., Forrest, G.C., Greenwood, H., Gardner, J.S., Jay, R., Roberts, J.R. and Landon, J. (1976) Clin. Chim. Acta *69*, 387.

Odell, W.D., Wilber, J.F. and Utiger, R.D. (1967) Rec. Prog. Horm. Res. *23*, 47.

Odell, W.D. (1978) *in*: Radioimmunoassay and Related Procedures in Medicine 1977, vol. I, pp. 3–39, International Atomic Energy Agency, Vienna.

Olsson, T., Brunius, G., Carlsson, H.E. and Thore, A. (1979) J. Immunol. Methods *25*, 127.

Orskov, H. (1967) Scand. J. Clin. Lab. Invest. *20*, 297.

O'Sullivan, M.J., Bridges, J.W. and Marks, V. (1979) Ann. Clin. Biochem. *16*, 221.

Painter, K. and Vader, C.R. (1979) Clin. Chem. *25*, 797.

Petersen, M.A. and Swerdloff, R.S. (1979) Clin. Chem. *25*, 1239.

Porter, R.R. (1959) Biochem. J. *73*, 119.

Post, K.G., Roy, A.K., Cederquist, L.L. and Saxena, B.B. (1980) J. Clin. Endocrinol. Metab. *50*, 169.

Pratt, J.J. (1978) Clin. Chem. *24*, 1869.

Pratt, J.J., Woldring, M.G., Boonman, R. and Bosman, W. (1979) Eur. J. Nuclear Med. *4*, 171.

Preedy, J.R.K. and Aitken, E.H. (1961) J. Biol. Chem. *236*, 1297.

Ratcliffe, J.G. (1974) Brit. Med. Bull. *30*, 32.

Ratter, S.J., Lowry, P.J., Besser, G.M. and Rees, L.H. (1980) J. Endocrinol. *85*, 359.

Redshaw, M.R. and Lynch, S.S. (1974) J. Endocrinol. *60*, 527.

Rees, L.H. (1976) Clin. Endocrinol. *5*, 3635.

Rees, L.H., Cook, D.M., Kendall, J.W., Allen, C.F., Kramer, R.M., Ratcliffe, J.G. and Knight, R.A. (1971) Endocrinology *89*, 254.

Rees, L.H., Ratcliffe, J.G., Besser, G.M., Kramer, R.M., Landon, J. and Chayen, J. (1973) Nature New Biol. *241*, 84.

Richardson, J.M., Steinetz, L.L., Deutscher, S.B., Bookless, W.A. and Schmelzinger, W.L. (1979) Anal. Biochem. *97*, 17.

Roberts, R., Parker, C.W. and Sobell, B.E. (1977) Lancet *ii*, 319.

Rodbard, D. (1971) *in*: Principles of Competitive Protein Binding Assays (Odell, W.D. and Daughaday, W.H. eds) p. 204, Lippincott, Philadelphia PA.

Rodbard, D. and Lewald, J.E. (1970) Acta Endocrinol. (København) Suppl. *147*, 79.

Rodbard, D. (1978) *in*: Radioimmunoassay and Related Procedures in Medicine 1977, vol. II, p. 21, International Atomic Energy Agency, Vienna.

Rolleri, E., Zannino, M., Orlandini, S. and Malvano, R. (1976) Clin. Chim. Acta 66, 319.

Rosa, U., Scasselati, G.A., Pennisi, F., Riccioni, N., Gianoni, P. and Giordani, R. (1964) Biochim. Biophys. Acta 86, 519.

Rosner, W. (1972) J. Clin. Endocr. Metab. 34, 983.

Rosselin, G., Assan, R., Yalow, R.S. and Berson, S.A. (1969) Nature 212, 355.

Rowell, F.J., Paxton, J.W., Aitken, S.M. and Ratcliffe, J.G. (1979) J. Immunol. Methods 27, 363.

Rubenstein, K., Schneider, R. and Ullman, E. (1972) Biochem. Biophys. Res. Commun. 47, 846.

Samols, E.C. and Bilkus, D. (1963) Proc. Soc. Exp. Biol. Med. 115, 89.

Scharpe, E.L., Cooreman, W.M., Blomme, W.J. and Laekeman, G.M. (1976) Clin. Chem. 22, 733.

Schoneshofer, M., Fenner, A. and Dulce, H.J. (1981) J. Steroid Biochem. 14, 377.

Schroeder, H.R., Yeager, F.M., Boguslaski, R.C. and Vogelhut, P.O. (1979) J. Immunol. Methods 25, 275.

Sela, M. (1969) Science 166, 1365.

Shane, B., Tamura, T. and Stokstad, E.L.R. (1980) Clin. Chim. Acta 100, 13.

Shaw, E.J., Watson, R.A.A. and Smith, D.S. (1977) Eur. J. Drug Metab. Pharmacokin. 4, 191.

Shaw, E.J., Watson, R.A.A., Landon, J. and Smith, D.S. (1977) J. Clin. Pathol. 30, 526.

Sigel, M.B., Vanderlaan, W.P., Vanderlaan, E.F. and Lewis, U.J. (1980) Endocrinology 106, 92.

Silver, M.R., Yoi, O.O.M., Austen, K.F. and Spragg, J. (1980) J. Immunol. 124, 1551.

Sinosich, M. and Chard, T. (1979) Ann. Clin. Biochem. 16, 334.

Sippell, W.G., Bidlingmaier, F. and Knorr, D. (1978) in: Radioimmunoassay and Related Procedures in Medicine 1977, vol. I, p. 229, International Atomic Energy Agency, Vienna.

Sizaret, P. and Esteve, J. (1980) J. Immunol. Methods 34, 79.

Smith, D.S. (1977) FEBS Lett. 77, 25.

Soini, E. and Hemmila, I. (1979) Clin. Chem. 25, 353.

Soll, A.H., Hahn, C.R. and Neville, D.M. (1975) J. Clin. Invest. 56, 769.

Stahl, E. (ed) (1969) Thin-Layer Chromatography (English edn), Springer-Verlag, Berlin, New York.

Steiner, D.F., Hallund, O., Rubenstein, A.H., Cho, S. and Bayliss, C. (1968) Diabetes 17, 725.

Sterling, K. and Hegedus, A. (1962) J. Clin. Invest. 41, 1031.

Storring, P.L., Gaines, Das, R.E., Tiplady, R.J., Stenning, B.E. and Mistry, Y. (1980) J. Endocrinol. 85, 533.

Storring, P.L., Zaidi, A.A., Mistry, Y.G., Fröysa, B., Stenning, B.E. and Diczfalusy, E. (1981) J. Endocrinol. *91*, 353.

Sun, L. and Spiehler, V. (1976) Clin. Chem. *22*, 2029.

Sykes, A.E. and Chard, T. (1980) Clin. Chem. 26, 1224.

Tantchou, J.K. and Slaunwhite, W.R. (1979) Prep. Biochem. *9*, 379.

Tengerdy, R.P. (1965) J. Lab. Clin. Med. *65*, 859.

Thomas, K. and Ferrin, J. (1968) J. Clin. Endocr. Metab. *28*, 1667.

Thorell, J.J. and Johansson, B.G. (1971) Biochim. Biophys. Acta *251*, 363.

Thorell, J.I. and Holmstrom, B. (1976) J. Endocrinol. *70*, 335.

Thorson, S.C., Wilkins, G.W. and Schaffrin M. (1972) J. Lab. Clin. Med. *80*, 145.

Trafford, D.J.H., Ward, P.R., Foo, A.Y. and Makin H.L.J. (1974) J. Endocrinol. *65*, 44.

Tyler, J.P.P., Hennam, J.F., Newton, J.R. and Collins, W.P. (1973) Steroids *22*, 871.

Ullman, E., Blakemore, J. and Leute, R. (1974) Clin. Chem. *21*, 1011.

Ullman, E.F., Schwarzberg, M. and Rubenstein, K.E. (1976) J. Biol. Chem. *251*, 4172.

Uotila, M., Ruoslahti, E. and Engvall, E. (1981) J. Immunol. Methods *42*, 11.

Updike, S.J., Simmons, J.D., Grant, J.D., Magnuson, J.A. and Goodfriend, T.L. (1973) Clin. Chem. *19*, 1339.

Utiger, R.D., Parker, M.L. and Daughaday, W.H. (1962) J. Clin. Invest. *41*, 254.

Vaitukaitis, J., Robbins, J.B., Nieschlag, E. and Ross, G.T. (1971) J. Clin. Endocr. Metab. *33*, 988.

Valdes, R., Savory, G., Bruns, D., Renoe, B., Savory, J. and Wills, M.R. (1979) Clin. Chem. *25*, 1254.

Van Steirteghen, A.C., Zweig, M.H., Schechter, A.N. (1978) Clin. Chem. *24*, 414.

Van Weemen, B.K. and Schuurs, A.H.W.M. (1971) FEBS Lett. *15*, 232.

Van Weemen, B.K. and Schuurs, A.H.W.M. (1974) FEBS Lett. *43*, 215.

Van Wyk, J.J., Underwood, L.E. and Hintz, R.L. (1974) Rec. Prog. Horm. Res. *30*, 259.

Velan, B. and Halmann, M. (1978) Immunochemistry *15*, 331.

Vodian, M.A. and Nicoll, C.S. (1979) J. Endocrinol. *80*, 69.

Voller, A., Bidwell, D.E. and Bartlett, A. (1976) Bull. World Health Org. *53*, 55.

Walker, R.R., Riad-Fahmy, D. and Read, G.F. (1978) Clin. Chem. *24*, 1460.

Watson, R.A.A., Landon, J., Shaw, E.J. and Smith, D.S. (1976) Clin. Chim. Acta *73*, 51.

Weetall, H.H. and Odstrchel, G. (1976) J. Solid Phase Biochem. *1*, 241.

Wei, R., Knight, G.J., Zimmerman, D.H. and Bond, H.E. (1977) Clin. Chem. *23*, 813.

Weiler, E.W. and Zenk, M.H. (1979) Anal. Biochem. *92*, 147.

Wells, I.D., Allan, R.E., Novey, H.S. and Culver, B.D. (1981) Amer. Indust. Hyg. Ass. J. *42*, 321.

Wide, L. (1978) in: Radioimmunoassay and Related Procedures in Medicine 1977, vol. I, p. 143, International Atomic Energy Agency, Vienna.

Wide, L. and Porath, J. (1966) Biochim. Biophys. Acta *130*, 257.

Wide, L., Bennich, J. and Johansson, S.G. (1967) Lancet *ii*, 1105.

Wilde, C.E. and Ottewell, D. (1980) Ann. Clin. Biochem. *17*, 1.

Wilkins, T.A., Chadney, D.C., Bryant, J., Palmstrom, S.H. and Winder, R.L. (1978) Ann. Clin. Biochem. *15*, 130.

Wilson, D.W., Griffiths, K., Kemp, K.W., Nix, A.J.B. and Rowlands, R.J. (1979) J. Endocrinol. *80*, 365.

Wisdom, G.B. (1976) Clin. Chem. *22*, 1243.

Wolters, G., Kuijpers, L., Kacaki, J. and Schuurs, A. (1976) J. Clin. Pathol. *29*, 873.

Wong, P.Y., Mee, A.B. and Ho, F.F.K. (1979) Clin. Chem. *25*, 914.

Wong, R.C., Burd, J.F., Carrico, R.J., Buckler, R.T., Thoma, J. and Boguslaski, R.C. (1979) Clin. Chem. *25*, 686.

Woodhead, J.W., Addison, G.M. and Hales, C.N. (1974) Brit. Med. Bull. *30*, 44.

Yalow, R.S. and Berson, S.A. (1960) J. Clin. Invest. *39*, 1157.

Yalow, R.S. and Berson, S.A. (1968) *in*: Radioisotopes in Medicine. In vitro studies (Hayter, R.L., Goswitz, F.A. and Murphy, B.E.P. eds) p. 7, AEC Symposium Series No. 11, European Atomic Energy Commission, Brussels.

Yalow, R.S. and Berson, S.A. (1971) *in*: Principles of Competitive-Binding Protein Analysis (Odell, W. and Daughaday, W.H. eds) Lippincott, New York.

Zuk, R.F., Rowley, G.L. and Ullman, E.F. (1979) Clin. Chem. *25*, 1554.

Zyznar, E.S. (1981) Life Sci. *28*, 1861.

Zaidi, A.A., Fröysa, B. and Diczfalusy, E. (1982) J. Endocrinol. *92*, 195.

Subject index